Essiac Essentials

Rene Caisse's Herbal Cancer Remedy

Sheila Snow & Mali Klein

Newleaf

Newleaf
an imprint of
Gill & Macmillan Ltd
Goldenbridge
Dublin 8
with associated companies throughout the world
www.gillmacmillan.ie

© 1999 Sheila Snow and Mali Klein
1 8586 0057 X
Printed by ColourBooks Ltd, Dublin

Photo of Rene Caisse (p. 36) from John Newton's film "The Rene
Caisse Story" by kind permission of Olive Enterprises (Muskoka) Ltd.

A catalogue record is available for this book
from the British Library.

3 5 4 2

Contents

"It is so simple that I thought no one would believe in it"
– Rene Caisse, 1974.

Essiac has come full circle. Now, more than ever before, it has become increasingly important that the emphasis be laid where it truly belongs – in the hands of individuals in need, who can make Essiac in their own kitchen, using their own utensils, rather than relying solely on larger organisations and commercial companies for supply.

Introduction

*T*his book was written at midsummer on the shores of a beautiful lake in Canada, birthplace of Rene Caisse who devoted her life to the development of Essiac. Its direct purpose is to encourage and empower those who are most in need to locate and prepare the correct herbs in the same proportions as Rene Caisse used to make up her herbal remedy.

There is no panacea for all ills and Essiac should never be described as such. As the authors, we wish to state that this book has been written simply to present the facts according to the results of our combined research. It is not our intention to make any claims concerning the formula and we cannot and will not endorse any particular commercial product. Our personal experience with Essiac has enforced our belief that everyone should be free to decide for themselves whether the Essiac formula might be beneficial to their individual condition. We inherited, for a while, some small part of the Essiac legacy. In writing this book we are handing on the torch.

Sheila knew and worked with Rene Caisse during the last few years of her life and is a close friend of Mary McPherson who was Rene Caisse's friend and helper for forty-three years. Mali had never heard of Essiac until 1993 when she and her husband Greg found themselves having to deal with an enormous, inoperable brain tumour in the back of Greg's head. In response to his final wishes, Mali founded the Clouds Trust, a charitable organisation which includes research into Essiac as part of its programme.

Our experiences with Essiac have proved to us beyond doubt that passing on accurate information about the remedy and encouraging further investigation into its possible palliative benefits is a worthy vocation. At the end of the day, if just one person is helped and encouraged by reading this book we have fulfilled our mission.

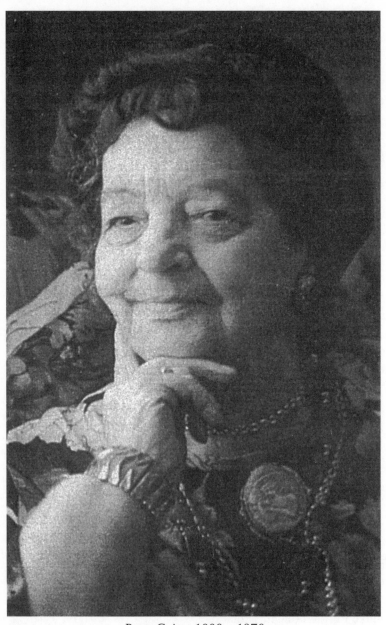

Rene Caisse 1888 – 1978

Chapter One

What Is Essiac?

*E*ssiac is a simple formula, blending four commonly available and prepared herbs to make a decoction. The formula was developed by Rene Caisse, a Canadian nurse, using a recipe originally devised by an unknown Native American medicine man exclusively for an Englishwoman with breast cancer in Northern Ontario at the end of the nineteenth century.

Essiac combines the entire dried and powdered Sheep sorrel plant *(Rumex acetosella),* chopped and dried Burdock root *(Arctium lappa),* the dried and powdered inner bark of the Slippery elm tree *(Ulmus rubra)* and the dried and powdered root of the ornamental Turkey rhubarb plant *(Rheum palmatum).*

It is important to note that Rene Caisse's Essiac is a decoction. This should not be confused with an infusion – a beverage made like tea by adding boiling water to the green parts or flowers of plants and steeping them to extract their active ingredients. By contrast, decoctions are very strong – unlike the weak beverage teas commonly sold in teabags. To make a decoction, hard materials such as barks, roots and seeds must be boiled for some time in a covered container. Throughout this book, Essiac will sometimes be referred to as "the liquid" or "the tea". This is because, when taken as recommended, one ounce of the decoction is mixed with two ounces of warm water to dilute it and it is then sipped as a tea.

The Essiac decoction is not difficult to prepare. The individual herbs are not expensive to buy and 180g/6.5 ounces of the com-

"When you want to extract primarily the mineral salts and bitter principles of plants, rather than vitamins and volatile ingredients, decoction is your method of preparation. Hard materials - roots, wood, bark and seeds - also require boiling to extract their active ingredients. Hard materials need boiling for about ten minutes and longer steeping to draw these elements out." - from The Herb Book by John Lust, Bantam Books, 1974.

bined formula will supply one person, taking Rene Caisse's recommended dose of one fluid ounce of Essiac each night, with sufficient for one year.

During her lifetime, Rene Caisse was a source of inspiration and hope to many, but she did not advocate 'lay' people making the Essiac formula because she said she didn't trust them either to make it or use it properly. She said many times that she'd have printed the formula in the newspapers but she knew that no one would follow it. Everybody would want to change it.

With Rene no longer available to verify and correct it, the Essiac formula has been subject to seemingly endless debate and escalating misinformation. Some of what was essentially hearsay has become passively accepted as fact. As a result, the way in which the formula has been interpreted has given rise to major discrepancies on both sides of the Atlantic.

Twenty years after her death and at the closing of the twentieth century, Essiac has come full circle. Now, more than ever before, it has become increasingly important that the emphasis be laid where it truly belongs - in the hands of individuals in need, who can make Essiac in their own kitchen, using their own utensils, rather than relying solely on larger organisations and commercial companies for supply. In the continuing quest for proven knowledge as opposed to naive and wishful belief, this book has endeavoured to set the reality against the myth, using the formula as verified by Rene Caisse's close friend and helper, Mary McPherson, in her sworn affidavit dated December 23rd 1994, Bracebridge, Ontario. Mary continued to make Essiac for Rene's surviving patients after her death.

Chapter Two

The Rene Caisse Story

*A*fter Rene Caisse had refined her herbal recipe she named it using her family name spelt in reverse – **Essiac**. Essiac is now well-known throughout the world as a healing remedy, particularly efficacious in the treatment of cancer. It can also be used as a preventative for cancer and for other illnesses associated with a compromised immune system.

Rene was born in Bracebridge, Ontario in Canada on August 11th 1888. She was the eighth of eleven children born to a French/Canadian family originating from Quebec. Her mother was the controlling influence on the family and was greatly admired and respected in the town.

"She and my father raised their eight girls and three boys to love and fear God, and to believe that respect and love of our fellow man were more important than riches."

As the children grew up, they became involved in the family business, married and had children themselves. Rene always respected and loved her parents, but she was very different from her brothers and sisters. Coming from a large family, she had learned to keep her own counsel and was very protective of her private space. Naturally secretive, intriguing and enigmatic, she was attractive when she was young, though never a conventionally beautiful woman. There are no records of any love affairs or

Essiac is now well-known throughout the world as a healing remedy, particularly efficacious in the treatment of cancer.

3

attachments and, by her mid-twenties, her genetic weight problem was becoming evident. She was intelligent and highly intuitive but growing up in a large Catholic family in a small town in Canada at the turn of the twentieth century meant that there would never be any money for a college education, especially for a girl.

Rene's Introduction to Essiac

Rene went into nursing, training in New York State and Greenwich, Connecticut, and graduating as a registered nurse when she was twenty-two. She was in her mid-thirties, still unmarried and working as head nurse at a hospital in Northern Ontario when, in her own words,

"One day one of my nurses was bathing an elderly lady patient. I noticed that one breast was a mass of scar tissue and asked her about it.

" 'I came out from England nearly thirty years ago,' she told me. 'I joined my husband, who was prospecting in the wilds of Northern Ontario. My right breast became sore and swollen and very painful. My husband brought me to Toronto and the doctors told me I had advanced cancer and that my breast must be removed at once. Before we left camp a very old Indian medicine man had told me I had cancer but he could cure it. I decided I'd just as soon try his remedy as to have my breast removed. One of my friends had died from breast surgery. Besides we had no money.'

"She and her husband returned to the mining camp and the old Indian showed her certain herbs that were growing in the area, told her how to make a tea from these herbs and to drink it every day.

"She was nearly eighty-years-old when I saw her and there had been no recurrence of cancer. I was much interested and wrote down the names of the herbs she had used. I knew that doctors threw up their hands when cancer was discovered in a

patient: it was just about the same as a death sentence. I decided that, if I should ever develop cancer, I would use this herb tea.

"About a year later, I was visiting an aged retired doctor, whom I knew well. We were walking slowly about his garden when he took his cane and lifted a weed.

" 'Nurse Caisse,' he told me, 'if people would use this weed there would be little or no cancer in the world.'

"He told me the name of the plant. It was one of the herbs my patient had named as an ingredient of the Indian medicine man's tea!"

The weed the old doctor had pointed out was Sheep sorrel.

The Development of the Essiac Recipe

Rene did nothing with the recipe until her aunt was diagnosed with inoperable stomach cancer in 1924 and given six months to live. With the permission of Dr. R. O. Fisher, with whom she was working and under his observation, Rene made up the herbal decoction and administered it to her aunt who lived for another twenty-one years with no recurrence of the cancer.

Dr. Fisher was so impressed by the result of the experiment that he asked her to treat several more of his hopelessly terminal patients. Some of his associates followed suit. One of the female patients had cancer combined with diabetes. Rene refused to treat her until she was taken off insulin because she was terrified of taking the responsibility for administrating the unproven formula in conjunction with a prescribed drug. As it happened, the diabetes disappeared first and the woman was pronounced clear of cancer within a year.

That same year Rene was asked to treat an old man whose face had been eaten away by a skin cancer and badly burned by radium treatment. His face was bleeding so badly that he was not expected to live for more than a few days. Rene treated him with a solution of Sheep sorrel and Blood root (another plant native to Canada) and the haemorrhage stopped within twenty-four hours. His face healed sufficiently for him to live fairly comfortably for the remaining six months of his life.

When Rene, at the doctor's request, injected her medication containing the eight herbs directly into the tongue of a man with cancer of the throat and tongue, there was a violent reaction. She later recalled,

"I was nearly scared to death! The patient developed a severe chill and his tongue swelled so badly the doctor had to press it down with a spatula to let him breathe; this lasted about 20 minutes. Then the swelling went down and the shaking subsided."

According to Rene the cancer stopped growing and the patient lived quite comfortably for almost four years without further treatments.

With Dr Fisher's encouragement, Rene began experimenting in her makeshift basement laboratory. Using mice inoculated with human carcinoma, she tested decoctions of each herb individually until the eight original herbs were gradually modified down to the four in the recipe as we know it today – i.e. Sheep sorrel, Burdock root, Slippery elm inner bark and Turkey rhubarb root. When isolated, the Sheep sorrel appeared to act almost immediately on the physiology of cancerous tumours. It was made up separately into a decoction and injected intramuscularly near the site of the primary tumour – i.e. it might be injected around the groin to treat cancer of the uterus or the cervix. The other three herbs were administered orally.

"Nurse Caisse, I will not say you have a cure for cancer, but you have more evidence of a beneficial treatment for cancer than anyone else in the world."

Medical Interest in Essiac Grows

On October 27th 1926, eight doctors signed a petition directed to the Department of National Health and Welfare in Ottawa asking that Rene should be allocated the facilities to formally conduct an independent research study to investigate Essiac. The Department of Health and Welfare replied by sending two doctors to have her arrested for 'practicing without a license'. When they found that she was working with nine of the most respected physicians in Toronto, arrangements were made for her to begin experimenting on mice at the Christie Street Veterans' Hospital in Toronto.

Dr. J. A. McInnes was supportive of Rene's work and arranged for her to meet Dr. Frederick Banting, already known worldwide for his discovery of insulin, at the Department of Medical Research at the University of Toronto. Armed with detailed records and statements, x-rays and photographs, she hoped this might be the opportunity to convince the medical profession that Essiac genuinely had merit and was worthy of further investigation. After a careful examination of the evidence, he sat quietly for a few minutes before saying,

"Nurse Caisse, I will not say you have a cure for cancer, but you have more evidence of a beneficial treatment for cancer than anyone else in the world."

He went on to advise her to apply to the university for facilities to improve on the research, even offering to work with her in his own laboratory there. But the offer depended on Rene revealing the identity of the full formula and didn't guarantee that she would be able to continue personally with her research. She also realised that 'they' would then have the formula which could simply be filed in the archives and forgotten, and her application to do independent research could still be refused. So she turned down Dr. Banting's offer.

Lacking the additional status of being a registered medical practitioner, she was well aware that she was in no position to be professionally recognised, honoured or rewarded for her work. And to be properly recognised was important to Rene. She had the willingness and the courage to research something new and potentially controversial but she was dealing with a professional hierarchy that was predominantly male and she was unprepared for the level of resistance and sometimes open opposition that she would encounter. Rene craved emotional stability and approval. When she didn't get it, she reacted in fear. Obstinate and uncompromising, with her back to the wall, she would attack rather than be attacked and for the rest of her life she held on to the one thing she knew she could protect – the secret of the formula.

The Founding of the Bracebridge Clinic

For several years Rene continued to work her twelve-hour shifts as a nurse during the day, spending most evenings absorbed in research and cancer cases. Inevitably the pressure of work began to take its toll. In 1927 she gave up her general nursing to concentrate solely on terminal patients. When tenants in her apartment building complained about the number of people lining up at her door, Rene decided to move out of Toronto to Northern Ontario where accommodation was much less expensive. She frequently returned to the city to assist doctors with animal studies at Christie Street Hospital and to treat recovering cancer cases with Essiac. Donations helped Rene to carry on with her work.

When her mother became ill around 1929, Rene treated her with Essiac, both in the form of injections and as a decoction, telling her that the doctor had ordered it as a tonic rather than revealing that she had been diagnosed with cancer. Rene's mother lived for another eighteen years and died in 1948, aged ninety.

Early in 1934, two Bracebridge town councillors, one a doctor, were so impressed with Rene's treatment that they encouraged the town council to allocate her the old British Lion Hotel in the middle of the town to house her clinic. The rent was fixed at twelve dollars a year, including heating and a caretaker.

Rene opened the clinic in Bracebridge in August 1935. She was forty-seven years old. For a while she was treating an average of four hundred patients who attended the clinic regularly once a week, lining up for their single dose of Essiac. There was no designated time for when they took it; they got it when they got there, regardless of whether they had just eaten or not.

As she testified to the Commissioners who visited the clinic in February 1939:

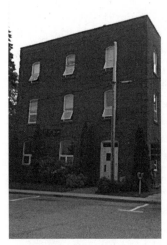

The Bracebridge Clinic

"*I have the patients come in and they register, and then they come into the desk and they give their history in their own words. They were asked to go to their doctor and get their diagnosis from him before giving treatment. In some cases they cannot get it, and the doctor absolutely refuses, and if the patients have been sent home to die anyway, I treat them on the off chance that I can help, but I have very few of those patients. You cannot turn them away when it is their only hope. In the majority of my cases I have the doctor's permission to treat, and the diagnosis.*

"*Then I have them sent to the treatment room, and I inject the* Essiac* *into their arm or leg or hip muscles, and I give them a glass of medicine, which is a blood purifier, and where there are open sores, I give them a local application. If there is haemorrhage, I give them a solution for irrigation to stop the haemorrhage. In cases where it is mouth and throat, I give them a gargle of my own making, and a mouth wash to cleanse. I would rather they use this than use any of the patented mouth washes; it is more healing I believe.*

"*There are a good number of the patients who do not need anything but the hypodermic injection. If their general condition is fairly good, it is unnecessary for them to take anything else or to use anything else, but there is little or no reaction. Occasionally, I believe, the treatment actually hits the seat of*

*Only Sheep sorrel was injected. The three remaining herbs were given as an oral drink.

trouble or contacts the seat of trouble, there is a severe reaction, because there are chills and a slight temperature. I say 'severe' because there are chills and a slight temperature, but not enough to be dangerous, but for possibly a half an hour or so, and it seems that after that happens the patient begins to feel a decided improvement. I find that in almost every case."

She had her sister and her niece helping her in the clinic. Other relatives were harvesting the Sheep sorrel. She was buying the three remaining herbs and making up the formula every evening ready for the next day. The Bracebridge clinic was open over the weekend for three days every week and she would be on the train going south to Toronto once a week to treat the patients there. For six months during the winter of 1936 to 1937 she was on the train again once every second week to make another overnight stay in Chicago to treat twelve patients involved in a clinical trial at the Northwestern University Tumour Clinic. Overworked and under tremendous pressure, she collapsed with exhaustion and a suspected heart problem early in 1937. The doctors ordered her to rest for two months.

She made one final trip to Chicago in early April before the study was terminated. Of the twelve patients, seven died during 1937. The remaining five were still alive at the beginning of 1938. To our knowledge there are no further reports relative to this trial.

Rene Caisse's Clinic Under Threat

By 1936, the Canadian Medical Association was intent on diverting increasing interest away from Rene Caisse and the Bracebridge Cancer Clinic. On July 23rd, 1936, Dr. Banting wrote to notify her that the Canadian Medical Association, under Dr. J.A. Faulkner, had 'requested' that he ask Rene to cooperate with him in setting up a new series of animal trials using the formula on mice inoculated with mouse sarcoma and chickens inoculated with Rous sarcoma. Clause four in the letter expressly stated that *"you will not be asked to divulge any secret concerning the treatments."* His empathy for the nurse was revealed in the sixth clause: *"If necessary, special arrangements will be made for the treatment of animals during Sundays and weekends",* the days Rene usually treated cancer patients at her clinic.

It was a clever move. By using Dr. Banting, the Canadian Medical Association were offering a well-known and respected name, with the promise of formal trials if she would transfer her attention from her human patients in favour of concentrating on animal experiments.

However, ten years had elapsed since their meeting and there had been no word from him. Rene now had definite reservations about dealing with a medical hierarchy that was predominantly male. Furthermore, she had already carried out extensive animal studies with Essiac, first in her makeshift lab and later with doctors at Christie Street Hospital.

She decided that, if Essiac were to survive, she had a better chance of keeping it within the reach of every cancer patient if she retained control over it herself, rather than turning it over to the anonimity of a big pharmaceutical company. When the time came, Rene wanted to be in a position to take an active role in the practical administration of the treatment. With or without assistance, she had to prove Essiac on its own merits.

In 1936 Rene was receiving recognition, which was important to her, for having the courage and willingness to research something new and controversial. She was also totally involved with the treatment of cancer patients at her own clinic and elsewhere. So Rene turned down Dr. Banting's offer.

Instead she instigated a series of petitions with the intention of delivering them to the Minister of Health and the Head of the Provincial Government of Ontario in Toronto as proof of support for her work and to authenticate her right to treat patients with the formula.

In answer to the petitions, the newly re-elected head of the government led her to believe that a Bill representing her right to practise would be presented to the Ontario Legislature as a Private Member's Bill. Frank Kelly, the Member of Parliament for Muskoka, and Leopold Macaulay, representing a constituency in Toronto, presented the Bill on March 24th 1938. The Chamber was well attended and the surviving cancer patients were well represented in the public gallery. The debate went on all day and made the evening newspaper editions in the city. Rene was correctly quoted as having refused to divulge the Essiac formula until the medical profession formally recognised it and her work.

Ultimately it all came to nothing. In line with a proposition presented by Harold Kirby (Dr. Faulkner's successor at the Ministry of Health) as a separate Bill to the Ontario Legislature one week earlier to set up a commission to investigate cancer remedies, the powers representing the medical interest put on sufficient pressure to advise a vote against the Bill. In doing so, they employed the usual delaying tactic of requesting that a committee be set up for further investigation. The government could not act without medical endorsement and the Bill was overturned by three votes.

For Rene this was the ultimate betrayal of all that she stood and hoped for. She was absolutely devastated and beside herself with anger and frustration. She felt she had been very badly used and deceived by people within the medical profession who had intervened in what she thought would be strictly a parliamentary matter. The Kirby Bill was ratified the following month to become law on June 1st 1938. Under the terms of this Bill, the investigating commission would have to be given the formula which should remain confidential. However, if for any reason it was accidentally divulged, Rene would have no claims in any court of law and could not sue them for breach of confidence.

From then on she felt continually under threat. If she did not divulge the Essiac formula she would be subject to a fine of between one and five hundred dollars. If she refused to pay she would automatically be liable to thirty days' imprisonment. She closed the clinic just before June 1st. Thousands of letters poured into the government offices from patients and their relatives, blaming the Health Department for the closing of the clinic and demanding that it be opened again. She was finally persuaded to reopen in August.

The pressure of the work and stress involved in dealing with a hostile establishment meant that, for her own sake as much as any one else's, Rene would have to close the clinic for short intervals throughout its active life. This time it had been closed for almost three months. The condition of a number of the patients who had been in remission had deteriorated and some of them were dead. The Commission was formally appointed later that month and Rene was interviewed during the following October. She invited them to visit the clinic. Two commissioners, Dr. T.H. Callahan and Professor R.C. Wallace, accepted the invitation for February 1939.

Questioned by Commissioners.

When Commissioner Callahan asked Rene about her current attitude regarding revealing the formula she replied:

"I still insist that I must have it acknowledged on its merit before I can give it, on the results I am getting. I think I am justified in asking that, Dr. Callahan. What do you think, Principal Wallace?"

"I am afraid I disagree with you, Miss Caisse," he said.

"I am perfectly willing to give it for the sake of suffering humanity without any strings attached, and I feel that I am justified in asking assurance that suffering humanity will have the benefit of it."

Commissioner Callahan replied:

"There can be no question about that, if it was acknowledged to be of benefit to suffering humanity, as any other case in the past in medical science has had the benefit of it. That is the point you need worry about least of all, it seems to me."

"I do not think so," she said.

The Commissioners stayed for one and a half days in Bracebridge, catching the train back to Toronto early in the afternoon of the second day in time for the rest of the weekend break.

The resulting report was sceptical, noting that there had been no clear verification by biopsy available for investigation.

The Commission examined her records and filed them for exhibit in the forthcoming Cancer Hearing scheduled to be held at the Royal York Hotel in Toronto on July 4th.

Approximately fifty patients were able to attend the hearing that summer, of whom thirty-five were summoned to testify on Rene's behalf. Dr. Benjamin L. Guyatt was the thirty-sixth and last witness to be called. Six months later, in January 1940, Rene was issued with an interim report which concluded that the formula had no merit. A final report was never published.

Rene had married her lawyer, Charles McGaughey, in 1938. Disillusioned and exhausted, she was fifty-three years old when the clinic in Bracebridge was finally closed in 1941. She moved away to North Bay where her husband had his practice. With his help she took out a lifetime patent in 1942 on another formula she had been developing in tablet form to treat prostate cancer and kidney problems. The tablets would be on the market until 1976 when the Canadian government cancelled the patent. She continued to treat a few patients surreptitiously with Essiac in North Bay until her husband's death in 1943 at the age of fifty-seven.

Rene would be under surveillance by the Ontario College of Physicians and Surgeons for the rest of her life. She moved back to Bracebridge and very little more was heard of her until she was introduced to Dr Charles A. Brusch from Cambridge, Massachusetts in 1959. He set up animal and human studies to investigate the properties of the tea but they were terminated in 1960 as inconclusive. A laboratory report dated April 21st 1960, which was requested and paid for by Rene, concluded that the formula was impossible to analyse.

She lived almost as a recluse, treating very few patients and remaining practically unknown to the rest of the town. She painted pictures and made beadwork for necklaces and costume jewellery. Often lonely and frustrated, sometimes bitter, Rene never truly lost her sense of humour and was not in the habit of openly complaining about her own physical problems. Mary McPherson was a long-standing and loyal friend who had played a major role in collecting signatures for the petitions in the 1930s. After Mary's retirement in 1969, she often kept Rene company during the evenings when her own husband was working the late shift as a security guard at the hospital.

Interest in Essiac Grows

Apart from some correspondence with Dr. Chester Stock concerning another animal study that had been set up at the Memorial Sloan-Kettering Cancer Institute in New York City, Rene's life was uneventful until July 1977 when *Homemakers Magazine* in Toronto published an article about her in its summer edition, entitled *"Could Essiac Halt Cancer?"*

Following publication, both Rene and the editors of the magazine were inundated with calls and letters. Rene had to have an extra telephone line installed to cope with all the calls. Primarily the article attracted the interest of The Canadian Cancer

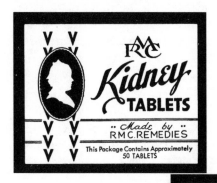

Rene's Kidney Tablets

The Proprietary or Patent Medicine Act.
No. 20027.

DIRECTIONS FOR USE
One tablet in the morning directly on arising with a glass of warm water. One tablet on retiring with a glass of warm water. Continue until improvement is noted when dosage may be reduced to one tablet each morning. The action of the tablets is greatly accelerated by drinking 6 to 8 glasses of water, daily.

Manufactured by
R M C REMEDIES   Box 485, Bracebridge, Ont.

Contents Patented in Dominion of Canada
under Patent No. 398359.

Research Foundation and The Cancer Institute in Toronto. Rene was cautioned not to treat any more people and an oncologist from Sault St. Marie, Ontario, was authorised to set up a human study for the formula using the cancer patients in his own clinic beginning almost immediately in August.

A small, almost defunct, pharmaceutical company based in Toronto approached Rene that month, promising to set up clinical studies on human patients all across Canada in return for exclusive rights to market Essiac. She was eighty-nine years old and at the end of a long and difficult life. She didn't want the formula to die with her but she didn't know how else to preserve it. Eventually she turned over a version of the formula to the Resperin Corporation of Toronto for the token sum of one dollar. Almost immediately she knew she had done the wrong thing but it was too late.

The promised clinical studies never got off the ground and the trials set up in Sault St. Marie were terminated in three months, concluding that Essiac had no merit. Properly conducted and focused clinical studies over a trial period of several years had often been promised but were never formally carried out during Rene's lifetime. Even the Sloan-Kettering studies were sporadic and not conclusive.

After so many years, she had given up counting on anything. As she said,

"My goal has been control of cancer and alleviation of pain. Diabetes, pernicious anaemia and arthritis are not curable but with insulin, liver extract and adrenal cortex extracts, these 'incurables' live out comfortable controlled life spans."

Rene Caisse - The Final Year

A public forum held in the spring of her final year at the St. Lawrence Market Place in Toronto failed to have the formula for the tea publicly recognised. In Detroit, Michigan, a Class Action lawsuit brought to court in a bid to recognise the formula in the United States in June of that year was dismissed.

Mary organised a big party in the Community Hall in Bracebridge for Rene's ninetieth birthday in August, 1978. In the following month, Rene was a great success and totally at ease at a cancer convention for alternative therapies in Detroit where she found herself among sympathetic people who understood and recognised her for her work in giving an important remedy to the world.

The following month she fell and broke her hip. She was in the Western Hospital in Toronto for several weeks. After this her condition began to deteriorate. One night in December 1978 she fell again. When Mary came by the next morning she could not get into the house. Rene was taken to the local hospital in Bracebridge where she died shortly afterwards on December 26th.

She had written:

"In my heart, I still hope and pray for a miracle but in my mind I only see closed doors. The disappointment is a tragedy that has made my last years sad and frustrating. I am grateful that God has given me the strength to retain my sanity.

"Perhaps some other country will have the courage to find and bring help to suffering humanity, though I had hoped that it would be my own beloved Canada, or our neighbour, the United States of America."

Rene Caisse is well remembered in Bracebridge, Ontario and Rene Caisse Lane can be found in the middle of town. The Rene Caisse Room, located on the lower floor of the local museum contains some of her original paintings, framed photographs, a glass cabinet displaying equipment for making and administering

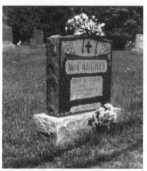

her remedy, and some literature about her life's work. The Caisse family plot in a town cemetery is in full view from the main highway and Sheep sorrel grows unchecked all over the site. The inscription on her gravestone reads:

McGAUGHEY
RENE M. (CAISSE)
1888 – 1978
DISCOVERER OF 'ESSIAC'

Chapter Three

The Essiac Herbs

*R*ene Caisse's original Essiac formula contains four herbs. This chapter details their individual characteristics and uses.

Sheep sorrel / *Rumex acetosella*

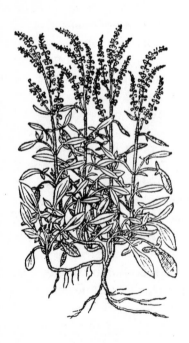

Sheep sorrel

A perennial belonging to the *Polygonaceae* or Buckwheat family, Sheep sorrel is found throughout northern Europe including Iceland and Scandinavia, in Canada, the United States and in the Drakensburgs of South Africa. Commonly known as Sourgrass or Dog-eared sorrel in Canada and Gypsy rhubarb in southern England because of the taste, Sheep sorrel is easily identified by its narrow, pointed green leaves ending in distinctive little 'tails' where the leaf joins the stalk. Sheep sorrel grows happily on neutral to acidic soils, on open heathland, under light woodland, some pine forests, volcanic wasteland and around rabbits. It prefers light and sandy soil but can be found flourishing on dense clay where the wetter conditions generally produce larger leaves. Unlike most docks, Sheep sorrel is not a hermaphrodite plant. Male (yellow-green flowers) and female (reddish flowers) plants are necessary to ensure adequate cross-pollination.

The stubbornly tenacious root system, once established, can survive forest and moorland fire, periods of drought and deep frost and is sufficiently invasive to eradicate many other species. That being said, Sheep sorrel will not tolerate either alkaline soil or being closely overshadowed by larger plants. The whole plant goes into hibernation during drought. Under stress, the chlorophyll content becomes significantly depleted and the leaves and stems turn red.

Along with the other sorrels, the herb has been used for centuries as a folk remedy as well as in salads and soups. The fresh leaves add a tangy, almost astringent, quality when used as a stuffing and cooked with fish. Medicinally, Sheep sorrel has been recorded as having been used to treat ulcers and cancer. Its action is refrigerant, diaphoretic and diuretic – i.e. cooling, inducing perspiration and increasing the secretion and flow of urine. Native American Indians have been recorded as using all parts of the plant, leaves, stems, roots and seeds, for both medicinal and culinary purposes. Both the roots and the seeds have been used to check haemorrhages because of their astringent properties. Additionally, the root contains four more elements to those found in the aerial part of the plant and should be included in a small quantity in the tea.

In her research Sheila came across this excerpt in Rene's files from a photocopy taken from an old book (source not noted):

"An old Indian doctor living in Oregon has been very successful in treating cancer by bruising sheep sorrel upon brass and applying as a poultice as long as the patient can bear it. He alternates this with a bread and milk poultice but always leaves the sorrel on as long as possible. This treatment is continued until the cancer is drawn out by the root. The writer

knows of two persons who were cured in this manner after their physicians had pronounced a cure impossible. It is also well to drink a tea made of the sheep sorrel."

*   *   *   *   *

Of the four herbs in the recipe, the quality of the Sheep sorrel seems to be the deciding factor as to the overall effectiveness of the Essiac formula and it was the one herb that Rene isolated during her early years of research as having a direct effect on cancerous tumours. It is also the herb which is most often commercially substituted in the tea as it is not easily harvested in large, commercially viable quantities. The cheaper dock plants, Broad-leaved dock *(Rumex obtusifolius)* and Curled or Yellow dock *(Rumex crispus),* are the substitutes for Sheep sorrel most often used by irresponsible distributors and suppliers. A packet of dried and powdered 'Sheep sorrel' could contain either of these – so be advised to check your source thoroughly. The dock plants share some of the same healing properties as Sheep sorrel, but not all of them. We have had reports of goitre conditions improving when Sheep sorrel is present in the recipe and deteriorating when it has been substituted by one of the docks.

Rumex acetosella has also been substituted by its 'sister plants' – i.e. Spinach dock or Monk's rhubarb *(Rumex alpinus)*; Sorrel or Garden sorrel *(Rumex acetosa)*; Turkey rhubarb or Chinese rhubarb *(Rheum palmatum)*. Sorrel and rhubarb are all acid or ammonium plants with a cell sap pH value 1.2 – 1.5 because of the large amounts of organic acids noted in leaves, stems and roots.

ANALYSIS
Vitamins: Antioxidants* A, C+P, E; vitamin B-complex (especially in the seeds): vitamin D; anti-haemorrhagic vitamin K; anti-ulcer vitamin U.

Minerals: Trace amounts of free radical scourging copper, manganese and zinc; calcium; chlorine; iron; magnesium; silicon; sodium; sulphur; trace amounts of iodine.

Other constituents: Antioxidant/anti-cancer carotenoids* + para-aminobenzoic acid, chlorophylls; organic acids as citric, malic, oxalic, tannic and tartaric acids; aloe emodin which showed 'significant antileukemic activity' when isolated from Sheep sorrel in tests conducted by the National Cancer Institute. The seeds contain manganese, vitamin E, and the water-soluble factors present in the vitamin B complex as pangamic acid (incorrectly known as B15), and possibly laetrile (incorrectly known as B17).

* *Antioxidants may alter the rate of occurrence of cancer and its subsequent growth through their action as anti-carcinogens, alleviating and protecting against damaging free radicals or reacting with their by-products..*

Burdock/*Arctium lappa*

A biennial belonging to the *Asteraceae (Compositae)* family, Greater Burdock *(Arctium lappa)* is distinguishable from the smaller *Arctium minus* by its solid, rather than hollow, basal leaf stalks and by its height. It grows up to 4 ft/1.21 m high with broadly ovate basal leaves that can be 15ins/38cm long. The large, globular flower head with its distinctive array of stiff hooked bracts, appears in July and August. Common throughout Europe, Asia Minor, Scandinavia to latitude 63° N, Canada and the United States, it can be found growing in pastureland, beside roads and ditches and along river banks, though rarely in woodlands. It tolerates both acid and alkaline soils, the roots developing well in moist, deeply composted earth. In Japan it is still cultivated as a vegetable.

The early settlers took the plant to North America where it quickly became

Burdock

well-established all over the United States and Canada, except in the far north. The native American Indians, particularly the Iroquois, the Chippewa and the Cherokee tribes, learned from the Europeans how to prepare the herb. The Cherokee made a tea from Burdock, Dandelion and White oak bark to treat varicose veins. A decoction of the root has been recorded in Indiana as a folk treatment for cancer.

Medicinally the herb is valued for its anti-bacterial and anti-fungal properties, for treating urinary tract infections, kidney problems, skin infections, arthritis and other inflammatory diseases. The high inulin/alantin content makes it particularly effective in treating dry and scaly skin conditions, and oil of Burdock has been used as a hair tonic to strengthen and encourage the growth of new hair. The plant is good for digestive disorders and can be used externally in a poultice to heal wounds and ulcers. Alternatively, diuretic and diaphoretic, it is an all-round blood purifier and painkiller, acting as a detoxification agent in the body, especially during illness.

The whole plant is concluded to be beneficial. The root and seeds are considered to be equally remedial, but only the root has been generally used in the Essiac tea. However we do recommend that some seeds be included in the decoction if they are available. Demulcent, relaxant and with a limited tonic property, Burdock seeds have also been used traditionally to increase the flow of urine, alleviate irritation and inflammation in the bladder and for all kinds of kidney problems, including dissolving kidney stones. They have a strong diuretic and detoxifying action and relieve coughs. Blood and plasma tissues, the respiratory, circulatory, urinary and lymphatic systems are all said to be positively affected by use of the seeds.

Studies by scientists at Kawasaki Medical School, Okayama, Japan have established anti-tumour properties in the plant as well as an antimutation factor, called 'the burdock factor', which is resistant to both heat and protein-digesting enzymes. A memorandum from a 1989 World Health Organisation meeting indicated that, under laboratory conditions, burdock was found to be active against the human immuno-deficiency virus (HIV). It is also a uterine stimulant and should be used with caution by pregnant women. The medieval German Abbess Hildegard of Bingen recorded it as being used to treat cancer.

The original recipe for Essiac uses six and a half (American) cups of Burdock root, chopped to the size of small peas. Although not a formally trained herbalist, Rene frequently used herbs to treat her patients and experimented with them in decoction. It was always her preference to use scales when weighing out her powdered herbs while using the familiar kitchen cup measurements for chopped herbs, such as the Burdock root.

Only the first-year root is used medicinally – i.e. taken from immature plants in which the inulin content is at its maximum level. In their second year, the plants have much larger and longer roots with a distinctive fibrous outer layer that easily parts from the more tender inner root. Depending on how they are cut, these two growth rings can be clearly seen in the dried root.

Fig 8 shows four samples of chopped Burdock root as supplied by the same distributor from a variety of sources over a two-year period. From these pictures you will see a considerable variation in the root's appearance, depending on the way it has been prepared.

Sample (a)   shows the root chopped into large and uneven pieces.

Sample (b)   shows the same root after shredding.

Sample (c)   shows the root peeled before drying and evenly chopped.

Sample (d)   shows the unpeeled root evenly chopped to the size of small peas.

When we measured the samples, using a standard measuring cup of the type commonly used throughout Canada and the USA, and then weighed them using conventional scales, we found some significant differences, i.e.:

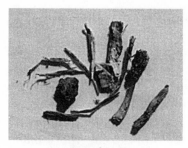

Sample (a)

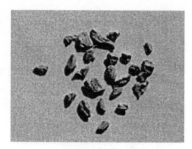

Sample (c)

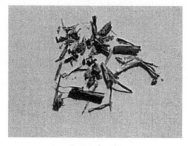

Sample (b)

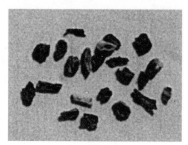

Sample (d)

Figure 8

6.5 cups of Burdock root cut to the size of small peas weighed 23.12ozs /655g

6.5 cups of Burdock root in large chunks weighed 17.5ozs/ 496g

As a result of the confusion over the weight/volume question and the variations found in the processing of the herb for commercial distribution, we have opted, for accuracy, to use weight when measuring Burdock root in the recipe given in this book.

ANALYSIS
Vitamins: Antioxidants A, C+P, E; vitamin B-complex.

Minerals: Free radical scourging zinc with trace elements of copper, manganese and selenium; chromium; cobalt; iron; magnesium; phosphorus; potassium; silicon; sodium; trace elements of calcium and sulphur.

Other constituents: Inulin, a nourishing carbohydrate containing sodium and magnesium that acts as a protective layer – the content may be up to 45% in the root in the first autumn of the two-year cycle and is anti-carcinogenic in that it has been found to break down the mucous membrane on cancer cells to allow the body's bio-defence system to penetrate cells; mucilage content can be as high as 12%; sugars; a bitter crystalline glucoside, lappin; arctigenin; benzaldehyde, a component of the glucoside amygdalin, the oily substance that has been credited in human studies as having significant anti-cancer effects; tannic acid.

Slippery Elm/*Ulmus rubra (formerly fulva)*

Also known as Indian elm, Red elm or Moose elm, Slippery elm is a deciduous tree from the *Ulmaceae* family and is native to North America, ranging from south-eastern Canada and the eastern United States to Florida and Texas. Preferring a rich, well-drained soil in the lowlands and beside streams, it can be found on rocky hillsides and limestone ridges but doesn't thrive there.

It is the smallest of the American elms, reaching a height from 40 to 60 feet with a trunk diameter between 1 and 2.5 feet. The trunk bark is deeply furrowed, grey-brown on the outer layer with reddish-brown underlayers, the twigs are a light red colour and rough to touch. A mature tree can be identified by the spreading branches forming a broad, open and flat-topped crown, and resembling the American elm's vase shape on the skyline. The leaves are characteristically rough and, measuring five to seven inches long and two to three inches wide, are larger than those of most of the other species. They are shorter on one side than the other. The upper surface is dark green, dull and very rough to touch, while

Slippery Elm

lighter and sometimes rusty underneath. Some people (Mali included) develop contact dermatitis after touching the leaves.

A log aboard a ship from England brought another more recent – and, this time, very unwelcome – colonist from Europe to North America. The European elm bark beetle carrying the fungal Dutch elm disease landed in Cleveland in 1930 and precipitated the greatest ecological accident to overwhelm North America since the Mayflower landed in Massachusetts in 1620. Ninety-five per cent of the native elms succumbed to the disease, destroying the characteristic appearance of southern Canada and the eastern United States, familiar as it had been to so many.

The elms are gradually making a comeback, but it is slow. We went from elm to elm in Ontario, feeling the leaves, examining the twigs and bark, and time after time all we found were young American (or White) Elms. Almost at the point of giving up, we were driving along a highway one evening, watching the most amazing sunset. The clouds were forming and re-forming around the sun, shot through with great rays of light fanning out across the western sky. A few miles further on, our driver suddenly swerved off the road beside yet another tree – and we found what we had been looking for in the front yard of a house just off the highway. Mali's hands and face were itching and burning all the way back home, leaving us in no doubt as to the authenticity of our discovery!

Ten-year-old powdered Slippery elm bark is sold as a coarse powder for external use and a fine powder for internal use. The inner bark was listed as an official drug in the United States and is included in the list of Canadian medicinal plants. Collected in the spring when the leaf buds are swelling with sap, it has an abundance of cells with a high mucilage content surrounding each fibre. These swell on contact with water, producing a lubricating or laxative effect when administered topically or by mouth. It is a cell proliferant, promoting rapid healing and restoration, and exhibits soothing, softening and nutritive properties.

The inner bark, extracted from freshly broken-off Slippery elm twigs, made a favourite chewing gum and thirst quencher in the frontier days. An early American ethno-botanist observed the Native American Indians, pioneers and settlers of the West using the bark internally for urinary and bowel complaints, scurvy, diarrhoea, dysentery, cholera infantum, and as a nutritious food. Externally it was used to treat ulcers, tumours, swellings, boils, abscesses, chilblains, burns and sores. The powdered bark was added to rendered animal fat to keep it from going rancid, while soaked strips of the bark were wrapped around meats to preserve them.

Native American Indians used the bark to make tea to ease fevers and colds, to treat bowel complaints and for pregnant women in labour. Mixed with milk or water, it made an easily digestible food for newly weaned babies and for treating stomach ulcers. The Ojibwe made a tea from the herb to treat sore throats. Both Indians and settlers used the outer bark to make ropes and baskets.

In some states in the United States, local law does not allow the harvested bark pieces to be any longer than 1.5ins in length to discourage the old Native American Indian practice of inserting them into the cervix to induce abortion.

ANALYSIS
Vitamins: Antioxidants A, C+P; predominant source of vitamin B-complex in the tea; anti-haemorrhagic vitamin K.

Minerals: Free radical scourging manganese, selenium and trace elements of zinc; calcium; sodium; chromium; trace elements iron; phosphorus; silicon.

Other constituents: High mucilaginous content; organic acid as gallic acid; phenols (including antioxidant tannins); starches; sugars; beta-sitosterol and a polysaccharide, both of which have shown "significant activity" (Pettit, G.R. *et al.*, *Antineoplastic agents)*.

Turkey Rhubarb/*Rheum palmatum*

A handsome ornamental perennial from the *Polygonaceae* family originating from the mountains of western China and

Tibet, Turkey rhubarb or Chinese rhubarb grows up to 8ft/2.43m high when in flower and thrives in deep, moist soil, in full sun or partial shade. Growth begins early in March, the creamy flower clusters appearing on the distinctive stalk in May. An innocent little plant with three leaves in an eight inch pot bought in the beginning of May at the Royal Horticultural Society's Garden in Wisley, UK was planted in a small converted vegetable plot in southern England. It became a magnificent specimen measuring 5' high x 5'11" wide x 3' deep (152 x 180 x 91cms) at the end of the following July. Fourteen leaves sprouted in three months, nine of them averaging 2' 6" x 2'10" (76 x 86cms).

Turkey Rhubarb

Rhubarb was one of the first plants to be imported from Europe to North America. Already familiar across Asia and Asia Minor, this species was the first true rhubarb to be introduced into Britain when Dr. James Mounsey from Trailflat, Dumfriesshire brought the seeds of both *Rheum palmatum* and *Rheum rhaponticum* back to Scotland after his resignation from the Russian Imperial Court in 1762. He gave them to the Professor of Botany at Edinburgh University. Of the two, *Rheum palmatum* has proved the most difficult to grow in England, being liable to root rot. However a single root dug from a six-year-old plant can weigh as much as 36 pounds.

Known to both ancient Chinese and Greek physicians, medicinally the plant has been recorded as containing both astringent and laxative properties, having a truly cleansing action on the gut and then acting as an astringent with its antiseptic properties. More recent studies have shown potential antimicrobial, anti-inflammatory, antibacterial and diuretic properties and extracts have been used to treat bleeding of the upper digestive tract. *Rheum palmatum* "has been demonstrated to have anti-tumour activity in the sarcoma 37 test system" (Beckin, M & Fitzgerald, D, *Tumour Damaging Capacity of Plant Materials*, N.C.I., 1952)

The leaves and stems of this species are *not* edible – only the root is used in Essiac. Turkey rhubarb is not only medicinally more potent but has a much less bitter taste than the medicinally milder domestic rhubarb roots (*Rheum rhaponticum*) which Rene used when she first began experimenting with the recipe, until she discovered that the Turkey rhubarb root was easily available commercially and easy to grind into powder. The roots of *Rheum rhaponticum* contain rhaponticin, a glycoside which exerts a hormonal effect on humans and should be used with caution.

The toxicity of rhubarb leaves of both species was once thought to be due to their high oxalate content but now it is thought to be due mainly to the high anthraquinone glycoside content of the leaves. In comparison, the roots display a lower oxalate and anthraquinone glycoside content.

ANALYSIS

Vitamins: Antioxidants A and C + P; some of the vitamin B-complex.

Minerals: Free radical scourging copper, manganese, zinc; calcium; chlorine; iodine; iron; magnesium; phosphorus; potassium; silicon; sodium; sulphur.

Other constituents: Organic acids such as gallic, malic, oxalic and tannic acids present; significant proportions of antioxidant anthraquinone glycosides which act as laxatives – including rhein, chrysphanic acid, rheochrysidin; aloe-emodin and catechins. Note: rhein has been shown to be effective in inhibiting the growth of disease-causing bacteria in the intestine and in treating the fungal Candida albicans. Rhein, aloe-emodin and catechins have all shown anti-tumour activity in some animal test systems. Pregnant and nursing women should not use anthraquinone laxatives.

Chapter Four

Preparing Essiac

M any variations on Rene Caisse's Essiac recipe have appeared in the years following her death. We give the recipe as verified by her trusted friend, Mary McPherson.

Mary McPherson first met Rene when her mother was diagnosed with secondary cancer in 1935. Mary also collected signatures for the petitions gathered in support of Rene. Both she and her husband were successfully treated for cancer with Essiac in the 1940s. Always a loyal friend, she became a regular visitor at Rene's home after her retirement in 1969.

When the *Homemakers* magazine article about Essiac was published, life became hectic for Rene. All sorts of people started calling her and dropping by at her house. When Rene was expecting someone, she would call Mary who would come over and stand guard in the kitchen keeping an eye on things while the visitors were talking to Rene in the sitting room. Sometimes two or three people would visit together and one would keep Rene talking while the others took a quick look around the house, searching for the evidence that might reveal the identity of the herbs that she put into the tea.

By then Rene trusted Mary enough to allow her to make up the tea with her. Rene would put the herbs into the water and Mary would do everything else, coming back the next morning to bottle it up. She visited Rene every day, quietly helping to ease the work load and no one ever realised she was doing it.

Mary is a very important witness to Rene's life and she has

been badly represented in the media by people who have never met her and know nothing about her. One article referred to her as a servant, implying that Rene would never have left the recipe to someone like her. But if Rene hadn't needed Mary, her friendship, her loyalty, her wisdom and her intelligence, Essiac may have just disappeared because she was the only person anyone could turn to for validity.

It is important to note that Rene always specified that three of the constituent herbs in Essiac, Sheep sorrel, Slippery elm bark and Turkey rhubarb root should always be used in <u>powdered</u> form, while the remaining herb, Burdock root, should always be <u>chopped</u> into chunks the size of small peas (i.e. petits pois) **Always question any mix claiming to be Essiac that doesn't comply with this.** (*see* Burdock p.21)

GETTING READY

Have all the equipment and ingredients to hand before you begin.

Utensils check list:
You will need one each of the following:

- Large cooking pot made from either unchipped enamel (UK), granite (USA/Canada), heatproof glass, or, failing all else, a stainless steel pot with a well-fitting lid. (We prefer to use enamel/granite).
- Stainless steel sieve
- Large heat-proof glass measuring jug.
- Stainless steel spoon for stirring.
- Measuring jug or cup indicating fluid ounces and millilitres.
- Glass containers for storing the tea – i.e. bottles with screw-top lids or preserving jars with new rubber seals.
- Accurate metric weighing scales.
- Enamel/stainless steel funnel (to prevent spillage when bottling the tea).

It is preferable, but not imperative, to keep one pan exclusively for making Essiac. Certainly when you are starting to make it, use whatever you have available at the time – but <u>not</u>

an aluminium pan, as the metal may be leached into the liquid during the making. It is true that Rene used an aluminium pot when she first started making Essiac, before she became aware of the adverse effects of aluminium – she switched to an enamel pan in the 1970s.

The water you use for making Essiac tea should be as pure as possible. **Do not use tap water.** Buy bottled, fluoride-free water with the lowest sodium content available, or use still spring water. Some people prefer distilled water.

There are still places on this planet where the water can be considered pure. Iceland is one of them. The tap water in Europe, Canada and the United States is subject to chlorination and sometimes to fluoridation which cannot be wholly removed by filtering.

Initially Rene used the local tap water to make the formula but, by the early 1970s, she was using water from a spring north of Bracebridge.

There are those who maintain that only pure spring water, as a living entity, can truly assimilate the potency of the herbs. We do not argue with this but we must point out that the water and the herbs have to be boiled together as a decoction for ten minutes and then reheated twelve hours later. Is living water still living after ten minutes at boiling point?

Europe relies on bottled spring water, whereas distilled water is readily available in Canada and the United States. This is claimed to be pure – i.e. free from chemicals, pollutants, poisons and minerals. Some people 're-energise and re-oxygenate' distilled water by shaking it well and/or setting it in the sun for a few hours before using it.

Sterilise all equipment used during preparation.
Treat the bottles/containers you use as though you were making jam or bottling fruit, <u>not</u> making wine.
There are several methods of sterilisation, including:
- heating in the oven
- steaming in the oven
- using a steam steriliser

- immersing in a large pot of boiling water on the stove (though this method is not advised for elderly or frail people who might have problems lifting heavy pots)

It is also possible to sterilise the bottles and lids using a chemical preparation sold for sterilising baby bottles. Carefully follow the manufacturer's instructions, rinsing thoroughly afterwards in freshly boiled water to remove all traces of the sterilising fluid before bottling the decoction

Do not use wine-making sterilising fluid, bleach or sodium metabisulphite for sterilising. These chemicals are very harsh and may alter the taste and content of the tea.

MEASURES

Liquids:
US/Canada
1 pint = 16 fluid ounces = 470ml
1 American or Canadian cup = 8 fluid ounces = 235ml
1 gallon = 3.785 litres
1 tablespoon = $\frac{1}{2}$ fluid ounce

Imperial/Metric
1 pint = 20 fluid ounces = 570ml
1 gallon = 4.545 litres
1 tablespoon = $\frac{1}{2}$ fluid ounce
1 teaspoon = $\frac{1}{8}$ fluid ounce

The US/Canada weight measurements in pounds and ounces are, for all practical purposes, identical to those used in the UK
US/Canada/Imperial/Metric
1oz = 28.35g
16ozs = 1 pound = 455g

The Original Rene Caisse Herbal Recipe
Bulk Recipe

Rene Caisse's recipe, as confirmed by Mary McPherson, contained the following ingredients for a bulk supply of the basic dry herbal mix :

US/Canada /Imperial/Metric
6.5 US cups/24ozs/680g Burdock root – chopped to the size
    of small peas
16ozs/453g Sheep sorrel – powdered
4ozs/113g Slippery elm – powdered
1oz/28.35 Turkey rhubarb root – powdered

However, for convenience, we recommend the following recipe which is sufficient to supply one person taking one fluid ounce/ 30ml of Essiac a day for a minimum of one year. It is not advisable to use herbs that are over a year old – please discard any remaining herbs from the previous year once the new harvest is available. This ensures maximum potency and is, of course, especially important when using herbs therapeutically, as in Essiac.

One Year's Supply, allowing for some Natural Wastage

US/Canada/Imperial/Metric
4.25ozs/120g Burdock root – chopped to the size of small peas
2.8ozs/80g Sheep sorrel – powdered
0.7ozs/20g Slippery elm bark – powdered
0.18ozs/5g Turkey rhubarb root – powdered

Total: 7.9ozs/225g dry herb mix

Preparing the Dried Herbs:
Mix the powdered Sheep sorrel, Slippery elm bark and Turkey rhubarb root together very thoroughly before stirring in the chopped Burdock root. This ensures that the Slippery elm bark and the Turkey rhubarb root are well distributed throughout the mixture. Place, well wrapped in a clean, brown paper bag, in a screwtop jar. Store in a cool, dark, dry place until ready to use.

To Make Approximately One Month's Supply of Essiac

Method:
Use the following proportions:

US/Canada
(if using a measuring cup)
2 fluid ounces (volume) dry herb mix to 64 fluid ounces water.

Imperial/ Metric
0.5oz/15g dry herb mix to 2.75 pints/1.5 litres water.

First stage
- Stir the basic herb mix in its storage container to ensure even distribution before measuring what you need into a small bowl. Immediately replace the jar of basic mix in a cool, dark storage space. Herbs deteriorate if left out in warm, bright kitchens.
- Heat the water in the pan to boiling point.
- Stir in the dry herbal ingredients.
- Reduce heat, replace the lid on the pan and maintain at a rolling boil (i.e. fast simmer) for another 10 minutes.
- Turn off the heat.
- Stir the mixture thoroughly with a clean spoon that has been rinsed in boiling water, scraping down any herbs on the side of the pot into the liquid.
- Cover and allow to cool gradually.
- Leave the Essiac decoction to steep with the lid on undisturbed for a minimum of ten to twelve hours – overnight is fine.

Note: It is important not to disturb the decoction during steeping time. Every time you take off the lid, you are exposing the liquid to airborne bacteria. Similarly, please don't put either your fingers or an unsterilised spoon into it to taste it.

Second stage
- Sterilise all the remaining utensils, including the lids and the seals for the bottles.
- Reheat mixture to steaming hot to ensure that only hot liquid will be poured into the hot bottles. DO NOT REBOIL.
- Allow the herbs to settle for a few minutes before straining the tea through a fine, stainless steel strainer into the measuring jug. Pour into the bottles using a funnel.

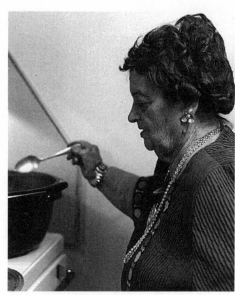

Note: Some sediment at the bottom of the bottles is quite usual.

● Seal the bottles carefully to produce an airtight seal.

● Chill quickly by carefully standing the sealed bottles in bowls of **cool** water. Avoid extremes in temperature as very hot glass is likely to crack when immersed in very cold water.

● After re-tightening the caps, store immediately in the refrigerator.

Rene stirring the pot of Essiac herbs

Essiac contains no preservatives. We advise that the bottled decoction is best stored in the refrigerator. Though properly sealed preserving jars will keep Essiac well in a cool, dark cupboard, all other bottles – in particular, those opened for use – must be kept in the refrigerator.

Dos and Don'ts

Don't microwave the tea at any time.
There are no short cuts to making Essiac and the microwave can never be considered as an option. All of its remedial value will be completely destroyed if it is microwaved.

You don't have to use dark coloured storage bottles/jars.
You can use clear glass preserving jars as you would when bottling fruit or any small jars that have sterilisable screw-top lids. When storing a quantity of bottles in an unrefrigerated cup-

board, it is important to ensure that whatever container you use has an airtight seal that you can test. Store in a cool, dark place, ideally where the temperature never exceeds 15°C (59°F)

Don't store Essiac in the freezer.
The potency of the decoction will be lost if it is frozen.

Don't use the decoction if it develops mould in the bottle. Discard immediately.

Like jam or bottled fruit, Essiac can go off early when:

- the equipment has not been properly sterilised.
- the bottled tea has been left to cool down for too long with the bottle caps loosely sealed.
- it is badly stored.
- it is left out of the fridge at room temperature for long periods between doses
- the dry herb mixture has been stored in plastic or badly-sealed containers in warm or damp conditions.

After use, the strained-off herbs will keep well in a covered container in the fridge for several days. They can be warmed up and used for poulticing as needed. (*See* "Topical applications" below)

Directions For Use

DOSAGE:
As a remedy for cancer:
Drink 1 fluid ounce/30ml Essiac once daily, diluted with 2 fluid ounces/60 ml of hot water. This should be sipped (like any hot tea), preferably before bedtime and at least two hours after eating. Food should not be eaten within one hour of drinking the tea.

As a preventative daily tonic and to enhance the immune system:
Take half a fluid ounce/15ml once daily, diluted in hot water as before.

NB: There is no need to exceed this dose.

"People will not stick to the dose I give. They'll decide on their own - if a little's good, a lot's better. That's the way they think," she said.

It is very important to use the dosage as Rene recommended, which was based on more than 54 years' experience. Rene was very concerned about this, which is why she personally administered the dose to her patients. The herbs are very potent, and in particular Sheep sorrel can have the effect of enlarging the tumour too quickly (see next page), so that it may burst, or a vital organ may become blocked because of its increase in size. Sometimes, the tumours will soften, dissolve into small pieces and be eliminated through the bowel or the urinary tract. Cancerous growths in the breast have been known to become encapsulated within six weeks to three months, and can then be removed surgically with little danger of metastasising in the future. Cancers of the oesophagus have also become encapsulated and removed cleanly and safely by surgery.

Depending on special circumstances, very occasionally in her later years, she would sometimes advise an initial dose of one fluid ounce twice daily for the first five, ten or (rarely) thirty days before reducing to one fluid ounce once a day. Rene was always very particular about this because she was aware that sometimes, when patients first began taking the Essiac formula, their tumours might enlarge suddenly as though they were gathering back the cancerous cells that had metastasised. When that happened, she either gave lighter doses or stopped treatment altogether for a time, to prevent a vital organ from becoming blocked. It all depended on the nature and position of the tumour. For example, primary brain tumours rarely metastasise and we have had no reports of this type of swelling when taking Essiac in these cases. *Essiac should never be administered intravenously.* During the early days of Rene's pioneering research, she found that only Sheep sorrel could be injected intramuscularly as an individual herb.

Essiac can be taken regularly, but you don't have to take it on holiday with you. If you have been taking the decoction for several months your body will not suffer from a couple of weeks without it.

Some people take it for six days each week, leaving one day free on the seventh. Other people, taking Essiac as a preventative only, take half the amount daily or one ounce daily four times each year (i.e. seasonally) for the two-week period immediately preceding the seasonal equinoxes and solstices.

Topical applications:
For lesions and visible swellings, apply the liquid externally once or twice daily in addition to taking the oral dose. Poultices can be made by putting the strained-off residual herbs onto sterilised dressings and applying to wounds that will not heal. It is also possible to use the diluted tea as a douche or an enema.

For carers:
Those who are most intimately involved in caring for a loved one who is seriously ill need to be well themselves. Taking Essiac as a daily tonic can only help.

Identifying correctly made-up Essiac:
There will be some minor variations due to the fact that you are using herbs which come from a variety of locations and soil types. Weather conditions are increasingly variable and the amount of sun and rain the plants experience during the growing season will also affect the quality and, to a more limited extent, the colour of the tea.

Those who are most intimately involved in caring for a loved one who is seriously ill need to be well themselves. Taking Essiac as a daily tonic can only help.

Colour: pale to mid brown, occasionally greenish if the Sheep sorrel has a particularly high chlorophyll content.

Texture: at the most, only very slightly viscous, similar to the smoothness that you might find in a good brandy.

Taste: pleasantly mild, with a slightly woody flavour.

Note: If any of the following characteristics are observed in the undiluted Essiac, it will indicate that the formula has been altered and that the tea may be in some way adulterated or not up to standard:

(a) very thin, pale and watery
(b) very thick and gluey, so that it is difficult to strain through a kitchen sieve
(c) yellow
(d) orange
(e) red and fermenting.
(f) very dark brown, almost black
(g) bitter tasting

Decoctions & Infusions

Please understand that Rene Caisse's Essiac is a decoction. Decoctions are very strong, and not like the weak beverage teas such as those sold in tea bags. To make a decoction, hard materials such as barks, roots and seeds must be boiled for some time in a covered porcelain or stainless steel container.

Sometimes the decoction will be referred to as the 'liquid' or the 'tea' because when taken at bedtime, on an empty stomach, one ounce of the decoction is mixed with two ounces of warm water to dilute it, and is sipped as a tea.

When you want to extract primarily the mineral salts and bitter principles of plants, rather than vitamins and volatile ingredients, decoction is your method of preparation. Hard materials – roots, wood, bark and seeds – also require boiling to extract their active ingredients. Hard materials need boiling for about ten minutes and longer steeping to draw these elements out.

An infusion is a beverage made like a tea by combining boiling water with the green parts or the flowers of plants and steeping to extract their active ingredients. The relatively short exposure to heat in this method of preparation minimizes the loss of volatile elements. Most often the water is poured over the plants, but sometimes the plants are added to boiling water, and the pot is immediately removed from the heat and steeped for a few minutes, with a tight-fitting lid to minimize evaporation.

Chapter Five

So Can it Help?

At least eighteen different types of cancers from the Bracebridge case histories are on record as having been successfully treated with Essiac

During her fifty years working with Essiac, Rene Caisse found that a variety of conditions, as well as cancer, responded well to treatment. Most of the cancer cases were considered beyond medical help by the time they reached her clinic. In the early days diagnoses were confirmed by clinical examination and by X-ray, rarely through biopsy, which gave some of the doctors the ready excuse, when people got well, that the cancer must have been wrongly diagnosed in the beginning. At least eighteen different types of cancers from the Bracebridge case histories are on record as having been successfully treated with the tea. These include cancers of:

the breast, cheek, kidney, pancreas, stomach, bladder, oesophagus, jaw, penis, uterus, cervix, ear, lip, prostate, bowel, chin, nose, rectum.

Many of the cancers successfully treated since 1977 are included in the list of early case histories. Others reported are cancer of:

the brain, tonsils, bone, ovaries, eye, salivary gland as well as lymphatic leukaemia and lymphoma.

Rene always said that she could not recall treating anyone with leukaemia, which suggests that it is more a cancer of our time, yet we know of two separate cases involving elderly women who both responded very well to Essiac. One had been given a matter of weeks to live when the cancer was first diagnosed. She lived for another eighteen months, enjoying excellent quality of life and using the time to hand over her work and business concerns to her family. The other lady has been using the formula for three years in conjunction with conventional therapies and is still doing very well.

Diagnoses involving brain tumours seem to be increasing. Depending on what and where in the brain the tumours are situated, they may not respond so readily to conventional therapies.

One interesting case we heard of involved a thirty-year-old man who was diagnosed in 1995 as having a tumour on the brain stem. By August of that year his face and neck were so burned with radiation that he didn't want to go back for more. He started taking Essiac that same month. In the September a cyst on his neck began to enlarge. It became very hard and sore and, by the end of the month, was leaking clear liquid and a cottage-cheese like substance. The pain around the cyst disappeared and by the end of October whatever was left of the tumour was discharging out of his nose. Subsequent tests reported him to be free of cancer and he was still alive two years later.

Other conditions listed in the Bracebridge case histories that responded favourably to treatment were:

Cysts, ulcers, benign tumours, chronic stomach and bowel problems, as well as goitres.

Women who have been prone to candida infections as a result of taking antibiotics have reported that they have had no recurrence of the problem since taking the Essiac formula.

We have had reports of people with diabetes reducing their daily insulin levels after some months of taking Essiac. Chronic candida problems have disappeared completely. Related to this, women who have been prone to candida infections as a result of taking antibiotics have reported that they have had no recurrence of the problem since taking the Essiac formula.

One lady in Canada sent the following report to Sheila in 1993:

"These are my findings after consistently taking the tea for five months:

(a) *I do not have aches and pains from my varicose veins. I also no longer experience the puffiness around them.*

(b) *I don't retain water as before and didn't experience swollen hands and feet throughout the summer.*

(c) *My energy level has increased.*

(d) *I have a feeling of well-being.*

(e) *I have lost eleven pounds to date.*

(f) *My eyebrows are growing in again, so very little pencil is required on them.*

(g) *My hair seems shinier and thicker and the roots are growing in dark instead of grey. – (Rene took a daily dose of the tea and retained her full hair colour until she died)*

(h) *A scaly psoriasis {eczema} patch at my hairline has disappeared.*

(i) *A dark sun spot has disappeared from my nose.*

(j) *I urinate more often and my stools are soft and very regular.*

(k) *My finger nails are stronger {no more flaking} and seem to be less bevelled.*

(l) *The small cysts in my breast seem to be disappearing.*

(m) *My gums are healthier and my teeth whiter. My dentist confirms this.*

(n) *My cholesterol level has maintained and my triglycerides have dropped four points.*

(o) *I seem to heal quicker from cuts and scrapes and pimples.*

(p) *I have not had gallstone attacks since starting on the tea."*

Dosage

Essiac seems to work better in smaller doses, adopting a more homoeopathic approach to the formula. Originally Rene gave each patient one dose of half a fluid ounce diluted in warm water once a week. That went on for years. Inevitably there were times when she ran out of the herbs. Then she would give people the dregs of the herbs from the last decoction, telling them to go home, add a quart of water and prepare the decoction all over again. And some people got well. She asked Mary (McPherson) to type out several different variations in the treatment, depending on the needs of the patient at the time. A lot of this happened after the clinic was closed, when she wasn't supposed to be treating anyone. It was only when the doctors connected with the Resperin Corporation started working with Essiac that Rene began to advise the dose of one fluid ounce diluted in two ounces of warm water before going to bed.

During the days of the Bracebridge Clinic she treated her patients *"once a week and in some cases twice a week. I like to have at least 48 hours between treatments.* For *"a good number of cases"* she continued such treatments for three months. *"Some breast cases if they are not too advanced, will disappear in about six treatments."* The patients she was referring to were being treated both orally and by injection. In this book we are concerned only with the oral dosage levels because we have insufficient information about Rene's injection methods and dosages.

Treating Children

It is difficult to offer specific advice about giving Essiac to children. However, the following case history could act as a guideline.

The parents of a three-year-old girl with an inoperable brain tumour used Essiac successfully, employing careful observation and familial empathy to decide on the correct dosage for their daughter's condition.

Two months after diagnosis in 1977 they began by giving her four teaspoons of the diluted decoction daily. One month later her white blood cell count was down to 3300 from 4000 and her condition was improving. They tried reducing the dosage to three teaspoons four months after diagnosis, but her condition did not respond well and she was back on four teaspoons, rising briefly to five for a couple of weeks the following month. Seven months after diagnosis she had put on 2lbs in weight and was doing well on four teaspoons daily, reducing to three teaspoons by the eighth month.

Ten months after diagnosis she was back to four teaspoons daily after a slight deterioration in her condition which adjusted after she had been taking the higher dose for two weeks. She remained on the four teaspoons daily for the next twenty-two months until her parents felt her condition had stabilised sufficiently to reduce the dose back to three teaspoons daily. Four years and three months after diagnosis she was taking one tablespoon of Essiac every morning. Seven months later she was taking one tablespoon every other day. She has made a remarkable recovery, thanks not only to Essiac but to her parents' love and willingness to observe and follow their intuitive responses to her needs.

Side Effects

When the recipe is prepared as Rene made it and her recommendations for dosage are followed correctly, only some mild side effects have been noted. Essiac is well tolerated when taken in conjunction with other conventional and alternative therapies, including steroid drugs – but should not be used to wash down other medication. Drink it separately to give its particular synergy every possible chance to work for itself.

However Essiac can have some side effects which might give cause for concern unless they are understood.

a) swelling – occurs when metastasised cells gather into the primary tumour.

b) cottage cheese effect – resembling curds and clear liquid, occurs as the cancer breaks up and discharges from either the bodily orifices or from localised cysts or swellings. A jelly-like substance can also be discharged or coughed up from the lungs.

c) more frequent passing of urine/defecation and other inexplicable discharges – occurring as the body detoxifies. If the symptoms are severe, with related nausea and pain, stop taking the formula for a few days until all the symptoms have subsided. When you start drinking it again, take half an ounce every other day, gradually resuming the original dosage. Remember that all diseases have a life cycle and a rhythm of their own, so follow your own judgement according to what your body is telling you about the dosage it needs.

d) aching 'on site' and headaches, linked to the detoxification process, have been noted as sometimes occurring when taking Essiac after surgery. Treat as for (c) and drink more water to flush out toxins from the body

e) fever or chills – sometimes occurring when the Essiac starts working directly on the cancerous cells.

Therapies which Complement Essiac

RED CLOVER (*Trifolium pratense*)
This is a short-lived perennial from the *Leguminoseae* family found in Europe and America. Native American Indians used the entire plant. They ate it and used it medicinally, externally in ointments for skin conditions and internally as a tea to treat skin diseases.

Rene told Sheila that this was one of the original eight herbs in the formula. She kept an old bunch of the herb hanging up near her furnace as a decoy to fool curious visitors into thinking this was one of the herbs currently in the formula. She would have tested a decoction of the herb along with the others during her early experiments, but abandoned it in favour of the synergy of the four.

We know of one case where a suspected carcinoma in a woman's breast disappeared in two months in the summer of 1977 during which she had eaten some fresh flower heads in salad and drunk a cup of freshly-brewed Red clover tea every day.

The herb has blood-cleansing, antispasmodic, expectorant and wound-healing properties and has been noted as containing four anti-tumour compounds including Daldzein and Genistein. The isoflavone biochanin A, an extract of Red clover, has been found to be a potent carcinogenic inhibitor. An extract, Uzarin, has been marketed in Europe to treat diarrhoea.

Jethro Kloss, author of *Back to Eden* recommends that *"every family should have a good supply of red clover blossoms"* and that *"the tea should be used freely and can be taken in place of water"*.

We would add a word of caution here. In large quantities, the herb could act like oestrogen; therefore larger quantities – i.e. two or more cups daily – should be avoided by women who have oestrogen-dependent breast and gynaecological tumours.

For all non-oestrogen dependent cancers – i.e. of the prostate, brain, skin, lung, stomach, colon etc. – drinking a fresh infusion of the flower heads up to three times daily may have a beneficial effect. Buy the whole dried flower heads, as opposed to 'rubbed' flowers (i.e. broken up flower heads). The herb should retain some of the colour of the fresh flowers and should smell distinctly sweet. Refuse to accept faintly scented, orange-brown rubbings.

Harvesting:
Only the flower heads are used. They can be gathered from May to November and can either be used fresh or dried to store for future use. They should be gathered on a dry day in perfect bloom and dried quickly to retain as much of their full colour as possible. Do not pick or use the fresh flower heads if they are already fading to brown.

Infusion:
Pour a cup of boiling water on to 1-3 teaspoonfuls of the dried herb. Infuse for 10-15 minutes. Drink up to three times daily. A little lemon juice can be added if desired. It is a good idea to buy a small teapot and keep it specifically for the Red clover tea. A small stainless steel teapot + tea strainer travel well if you are going on holiday and cannot take your nightly four-herb Essiac decoction with you. Red clover tea packs light and is not dependent on special storage conditions short term.

Some people take the decoction of the four Essiac herbs at bedtime to work separately overnight while the body is most rested, then drink the clover infusion as a refreshing drink to complement it during the day. As a strong tea, Red clover tea is very effective as a gargle and can be used four or five times daily. Fomentations and poultices have been used to treat external cancerous skin conditions and indolent ulcers.

ANALYSIS
Vitamins: Antioxidants A, C + P; vitamin B-complex as B1, B2, B3, B5, B6, B12.

Minerals: Free radical scourging copper, manganese, selenium, zinc; biotin; chlorine; chromium; magnesium.

Other constituents: Inositol: which is coumaric acid occurring as its lactone coumarin, a plant oestrogen, coumestrol, a naturally occurring germination inhibitor; glycosides – as a phytosterrol glucoside, a quercitin glucoside, a phenolic glycoside + cyanogenic glycosides (*"that apparently damage first those cells that are actively dividing"* and this *"had led to attempts to harness the toxicity of tumour cells"* – Simon Mills, 1991); antioxidant flavonoids; salicylic acid; isorhamnetin; trifolianol; essential oil; trifoliin; a hydro-xymethyloxyflavone, pratol; sugars including rhamnose.

KOMBUCHA TEA
This is made from fermenting a natural fungus or culture, essentially a living organism, with sweetened black or green tea. Kombucha originated in the Far East and dates back two thousand years. It has been described as a highly nutritious food drink, a potent detoxifier, an immune enhancer and effective metabolic balancer. We have had some verbal indication of benefits obtained from using Kombucha alongside Essiac, but no long-term reports as yet. (*See* "Resources and Suppliers" section)

VITAMINS C & E:
Some people have reported successfully taking supplements of Vitamin C from 500 – 1000mg daily with 400ius Vitamin E in addition to Essiac. In *The Handbook of Antioxidants, 1996,* Sharon V. Landvik *et al.* report:

"Based on cell culture and animal studies, it appears that

vitamin E and other antioxidants (i.e. vitamin C and the cartenoids, including beta-carotene) may alter cancer incidence and growth through their action as anticarcinogens, quenching free radicals or reacting with their products..."

SPIRULINA

Described as 'concentrated green super food', the blue-green algae Spirulina has a vegetable protein source of 65% – higher than any other natural food. It has one of nature's highest chlorophyll and beta carotene levels. Spirulina's total mixed carotenoids (natural antioxidants) equal 0.37%. Its naturally occurring blue protein pigment, phycocyanin, has been suggested as being active in strengthening the body's resistance to cancer through the lymph system. Easily absorbed by the body, it brings quick recovery from malnutrition and acts as a valuable food supplement in stimulating a return to a normal appetite during recovery from debilitating illness. It should be considered when undertaking a vegan diet to control cancer. (*see* "Resources & Supplies")

Animals

They seem to know what is good for them. Mali's mother's 14-year-old Siamese cat sits by the fridge every morning waiting for his 2ml dose of Essiac to be squirted down his throat with a plastic syringe. He was diagnosed with malignant melanoma, found growing as a small, blue-black lump on the back of his neck, in May 1997. He was dosed orally with the formula for four weeks and the tumour was treated topically once daily. It was successfully removed, the cat has continued with his daily dose and there has been no recurrence of the condition.

An old and ailing basset hound was rescued from the street on an icy cold February day in New York in 1995. The veterinarian found one large tumour on his belly, another on his liver and a third on his nose. He said that the dog had only a week to live and nothing more could be done for him. The new owner gave him Essiac and shark cartilage. Within a few weeks the stomach and liver tumours had decreased in size but the one on the nose persisted as an open, running sore which the dog kept scratching. His owner applied the tea as a poultice at bedtime, protective measures were employed to ensure that he could not touch the dressing and the wound began to heal. Four months later he was reported as being much better and very much alive.

A letter from Tigger's owner, Mr D. M. Canada, in 1994:

"About a year ago, our 14 year old cat Tigger started to lose the fur on her back and hind quarters. She became very unstable on her feet, which now seemed to lack coordination and she could no longer walk in a straight line. As her front legs started moving forward, her rear ones went in other directions.

"About six months later we heard a thump and found Tigger lying on the carpet, unable to get up after falling off her chair. We thought she was having a stroke because she stretched out her legs, rolled her eyes and moaned in pain. Since this occurred in the late evening, nothing could be done about her until the next day. Meanwhile the cat was somehow able to crawl into a secluded place.

"The next morning we were awakened by another thump. I got up, dreading the thought of possibly having to bury our beloved Tigger. I had some considerable trouble finding her where she had crawled under a bed. My wife, who picked up the cat and put her on the kitty litter tray, noticed that her digestive system was still working, so she decided to give her a drink, adding a few drops of Essiac to the distilled water. Tigger drank it. We continued to do this until, a short while later, she was able to walk again.

"Over the next two months, our cat completely recovered. All of her fur grew back and she never looked better. Now she plays like a kitten again. Today she was examined by a vet and her heart, teeth, eyes, ears and all her body parts are in purrrfect condition."

As a guide for treating animals, it is best to assess the dosage according to their weight. A cat weighing eleven pounds is doing well on 2ml daily whereas a large and heavy dog of 120 pounds would need an adult dose of 30ml daily.

Chapter Six

Attitude & Understanding

*D*octors differ as to how much they think you should be told about your condition. Some have to be virtually held to ransom before they will tell you anything, others will be much more forthcoming with a little encouragement. We have had reports of consultants and oncologists advising their patients to keep taking Essiac because of their markedly less severe reaction to the side effects induced by conventional therapies, all of which deplete the immune system and energy levels. One oncologist commented that he did not object to Essiac as he was well aware of the limitations of chemotherapy.

Illness obliges you to become much more aware of your body. You have little choice but to give it more than the usual amount of attention and inevitably to allow a whole variety of previously unknown people to give it a lot of sometimes unwelcome attention. That does not mean that you must immediately become a passive, acquiescent shadow of who you were before you knew you were ill. You are asked to sign the consent forms and so have the right to be directly involved in the decision making process. It is important to remember that your living and dying are uniquely individual experiences, and so is your illness. No two people are born in exactly the same way; no two people live in

We have had reports of oncologists advising their patients to keep taking Essiac because of their markedly less severe reaction to the side effects induced by conventional therapies

exactly the same way; no two people die in exactly the same way; no two people are ill in exactly the same way.

Seeing the Doctor – Keeping Control of YOU

All prognoses are purely hypothetical. A doctor's experience is limited entirely to other people's experience, not yours. You are in charge of you until your very last breath. You are in charge of your illness, whatever it may be, and you are in charge of the treatment. You are entitled to ask direct questions about your condition and the necessity and outcome of all proposed therapies, both in conventional and alternative medicine. As the parents of a dying child you should have unlimited access to all the continually updated medical notes. If you are considered to be sufficiently responsible to be kept fully informed about your child's illness, are you not equally entitled to be considered sufficiently responsible to be kept fully informed about your own?

Your illness is not failure. It is your greatest challenge, presenting you with the perfect opportunity to find out what your body needs and doesn't need. When you are first told that you have cancer, the chemistry of the disease is generally the last thing you have time to think about. All you want to know is how you are going to get rid of it. In that situation 'free radicals' don't mean a lot unless you are already a scientist or a doctor. Most of us are not. We find radiation or chemotherapy or a combination of both being recommended to us and we go along with whatever sounds the best, because that is what is available and we will take anything in the desperate hope that something is going to work.

The very word 'cancer' can conjure fear. Fear induces a state of semi-paralysis, mentally, physically and emotionally. When the doctor has a file with your name and 'cancer' written all over it on the desk in front of him, allow yourself time and space for the inevitable shock to register but realise that you do not automatically have to become a victim of that shock. At the end of the day, the disease is your disease. It is affecting your body and it is up to you to do something about it. The doctor can close the file, put it back in the drawer and go home for dinner. He is only affected by what is happening to you while he is reading the notes or talking to you during a consultation. You walk into his office with the cancer and it is still with you when you walk out. You are the one who goes to sleep with the disease and wakes up with it every morning. If you allow the very thought of it to eat you up, you will be eaten.

A little knowledge can help. Fear runs riot when nothing but passive ignorance is all that confronts it. If you are too sick and tired to want to know, recruit the energy and assistance of someone who cares for you to do the reading and the talking – and the shouting if necessary. Before you visit the doctor, make a list of all the questions you want to ask and take a cassette recorder and a blank tape with you to each consultation. Don't forget to take a pen and notepad. No doctor, consultant or oncologist should make any statement that they are not willing to have recorded. It is your life and your health they are talking about. If they don't have an answer to your questions, they must say so.

Your illness is not failure. It is your greatest challenge, presenting you with the perfect opportunity to find out what your body needs and doesn't need.

Chemotherapy and Radiotherapy Treatments

Both chemotherapy and radiotherapy kill normal and carcinogenic cells by generating the formation of massive quantities of activated and hugely destructive molecules called free radicals which may be routinely produced in small amounts by normal processes occurring within the life cycle of healthy cells. Produced in excess or insufficiently opposed by antioxidants and the scourging minerals copper, manganese, selenium and zinc, free radicals are believed to be associated with many damaging conditions including cancer, radiation sickness, rheumatoid arthritis and atherosclerosis. They are said to be promoted by radiation, atmospheric pollutants and smoking.

In *A Conspiracy of Cells, The Basic Science of Cancer,* Dr. R. Grant Steen states:

"Most cancer patients are treated with anti-cancer therapy that is often both immuno-suppressive and carcinogenic." [This includes both radiation and chemotherapy.]

No one tells you this when you are sitting dazed in front of the doctor, trying to take in what he is really telling you, only half hearing and then usually agreeing to whatever is being recommended, without being given time and space to think it through. In that situation you usually forget that you are allowed to think and that you are entitled to time and space to do it in. You do not have to be carried away on the momentum of the system which is programmed to launch you into one of several narrow channels of prescription and therapy. You have your own state of shock to deal with and often that of your friends and family as well, all at a time when you least need it and decisions have to be made.

Dr. Steen goes on to say that *"spontaneous cures are cases in which the body has rejected the tumour, in much the same way as a transplant patient rejects a transplanted organ. This suggests that the patient's immune system can occasionally succeed in killing an established tumour."* A strong immune system activates the body's natural advantage over radiation and chemotherapy treatment in that it can selectively eliminate the cancer cells while sparing the healthy, normal cells.

It has been recognised that the immune system becomes suppressed when the body/mind is in a state of stress. Within the immune system there are a number of different cells, each with specific functions. One group of these cells is programmed, among other things, to detect and to dispose of the cancer cells which are continually being produced as part of your natural bodily processes. Initially, the body goes into the familiar short-term, adrenaline-fuelled 'fight or flight' emergency response, shutting down all immediately non-essential functions, including the immune system. The chemical reactions released at the onset of stress 'switch off' the cancer-killing cells.

The chronic stress situation resulting from an ongoing, semi-paralysed state of fear and shock reduces the blood supply to the brain and diminishes the ability to think and respond positively at a time when positive response may be your only active recourse. Impossible as it may seem at first, it is important for your health and wellbeing that you resume control of yourself and your life as quickly as possible. You are only as helpless as you think you are. You have not lost the capacity for joy. Everything else is purely circumstantial. All pain, anger, disappointment and grief depend only on your ability to hang on to those feelings, to give life to those emotions, to magnify their reality. Even a terminal diagnosis is simply 'passing by'. Let it pass. Remember that you are still alive – healing can happen – and that it is possible to be grateful to the doctor who has presented you with a unique opportunity to grow in awareness as never before.

It is important to understand exactly why your doctor is recommending radiation and chemotherapy. It is equally important to know whether you are being offered the treatment as a cure or simply as a palliative exercise. You have a right to know precisely the anticipated outcome of such treatment. Just as you should know exactly what herbs you are using and the possible outcome of the effect they may have, you must know what you are accepting when you agree to radiation and chemical therapies, and you must know if you are about to become a statistic on a drug trial. You don't need to find yourself in a position where the 'cure' has become more life-threatening than the disease and, if you are not satisfied with what you are told, you should ask for a second opinion.

Similarly you should question the necessity of a biopsy and/or radical surgery. If you are being advised a course of steroid medication, you should be made fully aware of the side effects of such treatment. High doses of steroids depress the immune system and leave you wide open to infection. Steroids may make you feel very unwell and do you no good at all. At the same time, steroids can reduce tumour size and bring relief from pain. So find out why it is being recommended and balance the anticipated benefits with the inevitable side effects.

Persuade the doctor to let you begin on the smallest possible dose. Mali was told in 1993 by the doctor in the Veterans Hospital in Richmond, Virginia where her husband, Greg, was being treated for a brain tumour, that steroid medication *"swells up the face, gives a voracious appetite and puts unnecessary weight on the torso. It wastes the muscles of the arms and legs, causes stomach ulcers and rots the pancreas. In high doses it can also account for behavioural problems and is addictive. Reduce it too quickly and he* (her husband) *could experience withdrawal symptoms"*.

In that situation it would have been impossible to live with the brain tumour without the steroid to reduce the inflammation and relieve the pressure on the brain. Other drugs were prescribed to palliate the side effects of the steroid medication but there was no quality of life for Greg and Mali until they made their first batch of Essiac tea.

Orthodox Medicine and Alternative Therapies

A natural remedy made directly from plants will have a molecular structure that the body can recognise and assimilate as food. This does not mean to say that synthetic substances don't work but they are more difficult for the body to assimilate. Chemical therapies have been designed to affect rapidly multiplying cells. They will affect not only cancer cells but also other rapidly dividing cells, as found in the gut, causing nausea, vomiting, diarrhoea, and in the hair follicles, resulting in hair loss.

One of the new chemotherapy drugs available for limited use has been derived from a plant product from China. Its medical properties were discovered in 1957, but the crystalline substance carrying the anti-cancerous action was almost impossible to make into a solution until now. The sealed bottles of the drug are delivered to the pharmacist at the hospital, each with an accompanying leaflet designed for doctor and patient information. The upper third part of the leaflet is divided from the lower part by a serrated line and is designed to be torn off to be given to the patient. It is well laid-out in reasonably-sized print, some in bold type, and it appears to be informative and supportive, giving clear instructions on how to deal with symptoms and side effects. There is no mention of a desirable outcome.

The lower part of the leaflet is designed for doctor and pharmacist use only. The print is extremely small, not more than half the size of the upper part, and is written making full use of medical/biochemical terminology. The drug is listed as having been first authorised for use in October 1996. Under the heading *"Special warnings and special precautions for use"* – and highlighted for emphasis – the leaflet states that *"it is strongly recommended that the drug be administered only in healthcare institutions with adequately equipped facilities, including an intensive care unit"*.

Further reading of each section clearly shows that the drug has yet to be fully tested and that the side effects are expected to be severe to extremely severe. Studies in certain populations *"have not been conducted"*. While recommending that treatment *"should be continued until there is an objective progression of the disease or an unacceptable toxicity"*, the leaflet admits *"there have been no clinical studies to evaluate the drug reactions... with other drugs"*. It goes on to state that there is no known antidote for the drug and admits to two deaths as a result of its administration. An article in *The Financial Times,* UK, in March 1997 reports at least 94 known fatalities due to the side effects of the same drug. This is just one example of information that is available but rarely seen by the person on the receiving end of the intravenous drip.

Alternative therapies should not be considered exempt from similarly comprehensive investigation. Do not allow yourself to be persuaded that your well-being depends exclusively upon any one particular method or practitioner. Before committing yourself to any therapy you feel you would like to try, first make sure that it is not contraindicated for your particular illness.

There are a lot of therapists and practitioners. Many of

them have excellent qualifications and a natural affinity to healing, others do not. Be careful not to be pressured into accepting any that you don't feel entirely comfortable with and don't be persuaded into spending an enormous amount of money on treatments offering 'miracle cures'.

Be very selective. Check out the therapist's qualifications, ask how long he or she has been practising and the extent of their experience of treating people with cancer. Do your best to talk to other people who have been treated by that person and with that particular therapy. Check that they carry full professional indemnity insurance and politely take your leave of any therapist who suggests in any way that you have brought your illness on yourself.

Taking a Positive Attitude to your Healing

Whatever course of action you decide is best for you, be positive about it. Hating or resenting the illness wastes energy and you need all the energy you have to fight back. Don't feel guilty if you have concluded that a course of chemotherapy offers your best possible chance. Accept it and welcome it as a positive force for your healing. Back it up with Essiac to help palliate the side effects.

The same goes for radiation. Develop a positive and meaningful relationship with the machine. Give it a nice name, say hello when you get on the table and thank it when you leave. Drink your nightly dose of Essiac and apply it topically to alleviate damage to the skin and any scar tissue at the point of entry of the ray. Be prepared for the hangover effect from the radiotherapy which can manifest four to eight weeks after the treatment, leaving you feeling completely washed-out, with no energy. This so-called 'somnolent syndrome' will be self-limiting and will gradually settle down and go away. Those taking Essiac have frequently reported well-maintained energy and immune system levels, both during and after courses of radiotherapy treatment.

When you feel ready for it, ask the doctor the name and grade of the cancer and get up the courage to take a look at your scans. They will not be the most familiar or the most flattering pictures you have ever seen of yourself but, once you have adjusted to the images, ask the doctor to show you the problem areas. When you are back at home and just about to drink your Essiac, remember what you have seen on the scans and – **visualise the tea as a golden light surrounding all the tumour areas, soaking into every one of the cells.**

Don't be put off if you think you are hopeless at visualisation. Simply by bringing the thought to mind will be enough to make the conscious connection with the power of your own healing.

Without you and your illness, the doctors and the therapists, the drug companies and the herbalists would be out of a job. You are giving an uncountable number of other people a reason to get up in the morning and you are directly or indirectly putting their pay cheques in their pockets. They need you. It's up to you how much you need them. The informed patient has the best possible chance of survival and quality of life. We all have to die but let it be on our own terms and in our own good time. Unquestionably that is the right of all living beings.

Chapter Seven

Finding and Harvesting the Herbs – What You Need to Know

*I*t is important to realise how little you need of the four component Essiac herbs - only 8ozs/225g in all - in order to provide yourself with sufficient to make the formula for a minimum of one year. This includes enough to allow for some degree of natural wastage - i.e. inadvertently spoiling a batch by overboiling.

A good herbal supplier should be able to provide you with the correct herbs. However, not every herbalist or distributor can accurately identify the Sheep sorrel. If in doubt, talk to a qualified botanist.

Checklist:

- Buy the very best herbs on offer and organically grown if possible

- Remember that you are entitled to ask direct questions and to expect direct answers.

- National herbal organisations can usually supply lists of registered suppliers (See the "Resources and Suppliers" section at the back of the book). Call several companies and ask for price lists. Ask where they bought the herbs and how long they have been in storage.

- If the herbs have been imported, ask the country of origin and the likelihood of the herbs having been irradiated in transit.

- Don't buy the herbs in plastic bags unless you have no other choice. If you suspect that the herbs have been stored in plastic bags or plastic containers for any length of time, do not accept them.

- All food products have a shelf life and a sell-by date. Herbs are no exception. Don't be persuaded that herbs that have been around for three years are still as potent as they were six months after harvesting. They are not.

- There is a difference between wild *crafted* and wild *harvested* herbs. Wild crafted herbs are those that have been harvested from selected places and at the correct time of year. Wild harvested herbs could have come from wasteland around a landfill site at the end of a long, toxic season. Ensure that if you buy wild harvested herbs you get them only from a reputable dealer.

- Having satisfied yourself that you have the correct herbs, check them carefully before storing. They should smell fresh with no odour of mould. If they have little or no smell, they have been around for a very long time. Don't buy them.

- Store the herbs in brown paper bags placed inside screw-top glass jars. Keep in a cool, dark place that is completely free from damp or condensation and not near either a microwave oven or the electricity meter.

Seeds of any plant are a concentrated form of the multi-minerals, vitamins and enzymes of the mature plant. They are complete organic factors and we like to include both Sheep sorrel and Burdock seeds in the basic mixture for the tea.

SHEEP SORREL

Well harvested Sheep sorrel retains its green colour which is indicative of a high chlorophyll/carotenoid content, essential for the anti-oxidant qualities in the tea. Buy the dried herb either whole or chopped so that you can check stem and leaf size and the identity of the seeds. The leaves are curled and dry and dark green in colour. The stems are usually shrivelled and more pale. The seeds should be dark reddish-brown and the size of a pin head. Anything larger has not come from Sheep sorrel. If you find any seeds in the packet, plant some in the garden or in a pot and see what comes up. It is quite possible for you to grow sufficient Sheep sorrel for your own needs.

BURDOCK ROOT

The root needs to be chopped small to ensure even distribution throughout the mixture. It is kept in pieces rather than powdered to prevent the herbs from burning at the bottom of the pan while the decoction is boiling and to help keep the sediment down during preparation in order to produce a clearer liquid.

Burdock root is generally more easily available commercially than Sheep sorrel. However, like the distributors, we are always at the mercy of the methods of the growers because the root has to be chopped to size before it is dried. If the grower chops it evenly into pieces that will dry to the size of small peas you are very fortunate.

Sometimes you may find yourself faced with a quantity of rock-hard, large chunks and no other source of supply to turn to. At such times you have no choice but to shred it in a <u>commercial</u> food-processor before it can be used. Don't even try to shred it in a food-processor in your kitchen unless you have a very reputable and high-powered machine. Any other stands a good chance of being wrecked – and the root will look much the same as when you began.

Burdock seeds have the same properties as the root. As they are part of the aerial structure of the plant, we feel that they are important and should not be discounted from the recipe. It is not essential but, if available, some of the crushed seeds could be included with the root when making up the Essiac.

SLIPPERY ELM BARK

Buy the finely-powdered inner bark from a herbal supplier or from your local pharmacy. It should be a pale beige colour and evenly powdered. Don't buy a bag of brown powder. It could be anything. If it is fluffy with pieces of bark in it, don't buy it because you will not be able to grind it well enough for the formula.

Occasionally, unscrupulous distributors have been known to mix the bark with flour or willow bark. The resulting decoction is very thick and difficult to strain out.

TURKEY RHUBARB ROOT

Identifiable as a pungent, golden-brown, fine powder, it is generally readily available from herbal suppliers in the UK, Canada and the United States. Dull brown or reddish- brown powder is not *Rheum palmatum*.

Buy the smallest amount you can and specify exactly which species of rhubarb you need. If you are buying by mail order, ask what colour the root is and whether it is in chunks or is already powdered. If you have to buy it as dried chunks of root, you will find that it grinds down easily in a food-processor.

Harvesting the herbs yourself

If you decide to try to grow or harvest these herbs yourself, it is essential that you should be sensitive to the fact that they are destined to be used for human or animal consumption. Your herbs can either be wild crafted or grown specifically for the Essiac formula.

If the plant is not listed as a protected species, in most countries it is not illegal to harvest its seed and aerial parts from the wild but it is illegal to dig up established plants and roots and to destroy established colonies of the plant. Check this out in your own area.

Harvesting from the wild demands a great deal of care and

sensitivity as to the needs of the environment and other people's requirements. Only pick exactly what you need and take every precaution to ensure that the plant is left in a state sufficient to sustain its natural life cycle. Wild crafted herbs should be gathered from areas free from large numbers of people and dogs and as far as possible from roads, factories and regularly farmed arable land where they are likely to have been sprayed with pesticides and herbicides.

Herbs that are grown specifically for Essiac must be organically grown, i.e. planted in unpolluted soil that has not been, and will not be, treated with any form of chemical fertiliser or weed killer. Pollution is defined as contamination by herbicides, chemical waste, vehicle exhaust pollution, domestic animal pollution and/or artificial fertilisation programmes.

Remember that every variation in climate and location may demand improvisation on the basic theme. Good husbandry and good practice ensure a continual sensitivity to the volatile nature of the beneficial aspects of the herbs.

SHEEP SORREL

As there has been some doubt about the quality and validity of supply, you may decide to grow your own Sheep sorrel. Given rain and sunshine in good measure throughout the growing season, it is possible to take at least two, often three, cuttings from each plant from May to September. This will vary according to country, climate and locality.

In south-east England during a warm, dry summer on light soil, it is possible to harvest from mid-May to the end of August. Most of the plants are cut just prior to flowering but we ensure that some flowers and seeds are included in the overall gathering. Rene Caisse advocated using the whole herb and, to that end, in addition to the summer crop, a root harvest can be taken at the end of the year (November to December) using the opportunity to thin the plants in preparation for the spring growth the following year. Good husbandry is the key to growing and maintaining Sheep sorrel. As you can see from Growing Trial One on **page 118**, a small plot of one metre/39 inches square in the garden can provide enough Sheep sorrel for a minimum of five people for a year to fifteen months.

Scale down the growing area to suit your needs and your situation. If you do not have a garden or it has been heavily treated with chemical fertiliser or weed-killer, it may be worth investing in either a specialist grow bag to keep on the patio or balcony, or filling a large, well drained plant trough with lime-free potting compost. Avoid using peat, as it can no longer be considered an organic growing medium. Never fertilise the plants as this will encourage too much leaf production and perhaps an imbalance of nitrogen. Sheep sorrel is a plant that thrives naturally in light, well drained soil as long as it has enough water.

It is best either to plant seed in the spring or to transplant small plants in autumn or spring (depending on the possibility of rain) while maintaining a vigilant hand-weeding programme for at least the first two years until the root system has become firmly established and predominantly invasive. Sheep sorrel is tolerant of dry soil only once it is firmly established.

A small plot of one metre/39 inches square in the garden can provide enough Sheep sorrel for a minimum of five people for a year to fifteen months

The leaves and the soil must be regularly moistened for at least the first ten days after transplanting. During the first year after planting, bearing in mind that you want the plants to thicken and spread while they are in the initial process of establishing, it is better to harvest them lightly and not allow the plants to flower and go to seed. Do not cut close to the base of the plant when gathering.

Cutting:

Sheep sorrel is much easier to cut when there are large clumps of the plant growing close together, unaffected by grass or other plants, emphasising the necessity of regular hand-weeding.

On a dry day after the dew has lifted, cut well-established

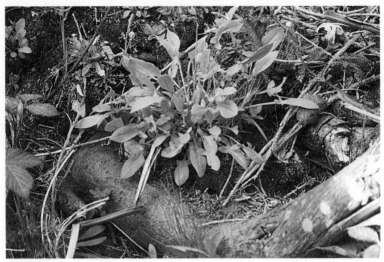

Sheep sorrel

plants to within half an inch of their base using clean, sharp shears. You should aim to have the plants out of the collecting bag and spread out to dry within four hours of harvesting. Do not leave the cut plants overnight in plastic carrier bags as they quickly begin to compost.

Drying:

Mali's years of making excellent organic hay for horses taught her the value of drying herbage as quickly as possible while exposing the minimum crop to direct sunlight.

Options for drying Sheep sorrel:

It is important that the herb is dried as quickly and as naturally as possible. The following guidelines will help you achieve the best possible results:

- Spread the herb out on clean cotton or absorbent paper in a warm, dry, dark cupboard, turning daily.

- Hang bunches of the herb in a warm, dark, dry cupboard.

- Spread the herb on clean cotton or muslin sheets, covered with agricultural fleece to protect from sunlight and lay out in

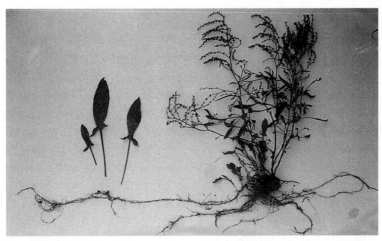

Sheep sorrel

a well-ventilated, shaded greenhouse. This is an option to consider if you are allergic to hay/pollen and don't want the herb drying in the house or if you have a large quantity to dry.

- Buy a small dehydrator.

It is important to remember that the herb needs air circulating around it and under it during the drying process. The cotton or paper should be spread over slatted wooden shelves/racks whenever possible. Do not expose the herb to damp or wet conditions during the drying process.

Storing:

Store quantities of the whole, dried herb tied up in unbleached cotton bags in a cool, dark and dry cupboard that has neither hot water pipes nor electric cables running either directly underneath it or above it. Ideally the temperature of the storage environment should never exceed 15°C (59°F). Pillowcases made from 100% unbleached, natural cotton make good storage bags. While it is important to minimise oxidation by avoiding exposure to light and air, the storage containers must be sufficiently porous to minimise any possibility of condensation damage during long-term storage. Equally, care must be taken to avoid exposure to pest attack.

Preparation for use:

We recommend that you buy and wear a dust mask while handling the powdered dried herb, especially when handling the root.

Coarsely powder the Sheep sorrel immediately before mixing it with the three other herbs. An ordinary food-processor will usually grind small amounts of the herb adequately. Process the Sheep sorrel carefully, using short bursts of power so as not to overheat the herb. The resulting powder should be green to dark green in colour and should smell sweet and fresh (similar to a summer-scented bale of perfect hay split open in midwinter). Try to use it as quickly as possible in order to maintain freshness. Only aged or badly harvested Sheep sorrel turns beige when powdered.

Cutting and storing the root:

Thin the plants by taking the root harvest some time after the first frosts, up to and until the beginning of January when all the life and energy of the plant has retreated underground. Sheep sorrel is very forgiving and will quickly re-establish itself the following spring providing the root crop is taken with care and consideration to leave enough of the main root system in the soil.

Try to harvest the root when the soil is as dry as possible. Shake off the excess soil before leaving the site. Wash the roots and shake them well to remove excess moisture. Dry as usual. Store in a cool dark cupboard. Powder as needed.

Note: The root is very potent. Do not inhale the powder. One level teaspoonful of it is sufficient for each 16 ounces of the powdered summer harvest of leaves.

BURDOCK

Root:

This can be harvested either in the autumn when the leaves have died down and all the vitality of the plant has retreated into the root, or in the spring just as the new leaves are showing above the soil. Wash and clean the root very well to remove all traces of

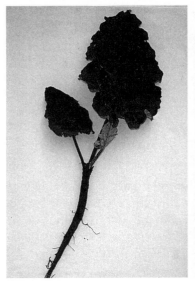

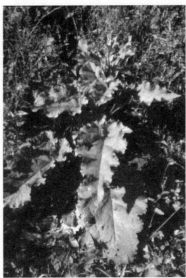

Burdock root   *Burdock plant before flowering*

earth and debris. Chop evenly to the size of small peas, bearing in mind that the root pieces will reduce by approximately one third in size during the drying process. Spread out on clean cotton or absorbent paper and dry as for Sheep sorrel, turning every day until completely dried out. Store tied up in cotton bags or in well-sealed brown paper bags. Use as needed.

Note: 16ozs/453g freshly harvested and scrubbed root, harvested mid-June as an experiment from four plants, dried down after five days in a warm, dark linen cupboard to 2.5ozs/ 70g. The roots will be larger and heavier with less water content when harvested at the correct time of year but this experiment does suggest that the roots of as many as eight plants might have to be harvested at a total minimum weight of two pounds wet weight to produce enough dried root for one person for one year.

Seed:

Bearing in mind that the plant is a biennial and will die during the winter after seeding, allow some of the seed to scatter and harvest the rest when ripe on a dry, sunny day during the autumn. Shake the seeds out of the 'burr heads' and dry by spreading them out on clean cotton or muslin in full sun. Store them as for the root, lightly crushing or grinding them to break the hard outer casing just before including in the tea.

Protect your hands when handling the burr heads, as the hooked bracts can cling as tenaciously to human skin as they do to fur or clothing.

SLIPPERY ELM

The method for harvesting Slippery elm bark is simple. Don't! Unless you have a large tree on your property that you have a particularly good relationship with and you are an experienced arborist.

The trees have suffered enough desecration by disease and careless harvesting. Buy the ready-prepared powdered bark and trust that those who are responsible for collecting it have done the job with grace. Once common in the wild, commercial interests – as well as Dutch elm disease – have taken their toll as spring harvesting of the bark can lead to permanent damage or the complete destruction of the tree.

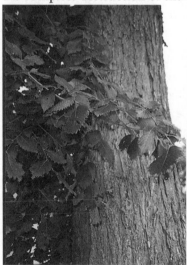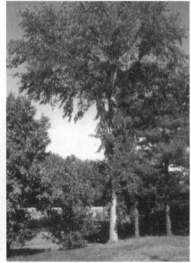

Slippery elm

Theoretically the innermost bark is stripped from a large limb, rather then the trunk, of a mature tree in the early spring when the sap is running. Stripping the trunk can, and often does, kill the tree. The inner bark separates easily from the outer part in one-inch wide strips that are two to three feet long and approximately a quarter of an inch thick. Good quality bark pieces are tough and flexible and bend without breaking. Inferior grades are brittle and snap easily. The bark is dried whole in strips and powdered before use.

TURKEY RHUBARB

Considering how little you need, it is hardly practical to harvest the root for yourself unless you have *Rheum palmatum* in your garden and the plant is more than six years old. The roots are not considered to be fully medicinally potent until then.

Treat the root as for Burdock, cleaning and chopping to size before drying. Powder before use, taking great care not to inhale the herb as you process it. The resulting powder should be a warm, golden colour. Put it, well-wrapped in a clean, brown paper bag, in a screw-top glass jar and store in a cool dark place.

Note: Make a practice of never leaving any of the herbs or the prepared dry mixture exposed to heat or damp conditions or under prolonged exposure to light during storage. Aim to use

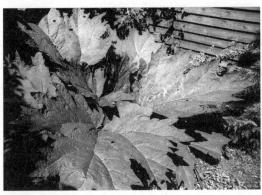

all the herbs in store within fifteen months after harvesting.

Turkey Rhubarb

Chapter Eight

Myth and Reality

*D*ue in part to Rene's reticence in disclosing details of the formula, the myths surrounding Essiac have become legion. The only way to get to the truth is to go back to the source and examine some of the more widely-held misconceptions and beliefs.

Myth: The recipe as confirmed by Mary McPherson is not a valid version of Rene's working formula.
Reality: Mary was well respected by Rene and was allowed to help make the Essiac during Rene's final years. She continued to supply the decoction to Rene's existing patients after her death. There was no deterioration either in their condition or in the quality of the Essiac. The taste was the same and they continued to return to Mary for further supplies.

A copy of the Essiac formula, as verified by Mary McPherson, is prominent on one of the walls of the museum in Bracebridge, Ontario. This recipe has been carefully and independently researched by Sheila Snow, drawing on her own recollections and research material from her association with Rene and piecing together information both from other people who knew Rene and from some of the doctors she collaborated with during the 1970s.

The final test was to examine and compare the colour, taste and texture of the made-up tea, all of which were found to be sympathetic to Rene's decoction.

Rene can be seen holding two clear bottles of the tea in John Newton's film, *'The Rene Caisse Story'*, the only known original film archive shot at her home in Hiram Street, Bracebridge, 1978 (*See* "Resources and Suppliers" for details of how to obtain this video)

Myth: An Ojibwe Indian herbalist gave Rene the recipe and instructed her how to use it.

Reality: There were a number of Native American Indian tribes living in Northern Ontario at the end of the nineteenth century including Algonquin, Cree, Cherokee, Huron, Iroquois and Ojibwe. The old medicine man could have belonged to any one of those tribes or he could have been a wandering seer from another region. There is no evidence to support the theory that the herbal formula came exclusively from the Ojibwe. In 1977 Rene wrote:

"I want this clearly understood. I did not get my treatment from an Indian. In fact I never saw a real Indian in my life."

As far as we know, Rene Caisse was the only person to receive and retain the recipe which had been freely given by the elderly medicine man to the original Englishwoman. Rene chose to develop and use it without the desire for material gain, reverencing the Native American sense of honour to the divine. Our personal experience with Essiac has continually proved the importance of retaining this sense of honour and respect in researching and handling the formula.

Myth: The Canadian government burned all of Rene's records after her death in 1978. Later it conspired to prevent terminal cancer patients from obtaining Essiac.

Reality: The rumour about the government burning Rene's records has been circulating for almost a decade. It did nothing of the kind! In fact, while relatives were sorting through her possessions and personal belongings, some of Rene's papers were burned in an oil drum behind her home after she died.

When terminal patients, now without Essiac, begged the government to provide them with the remedy, Ottawa's Health and Welfare Department gave Dr. M. Dymond of the Resperin Corporation permission to make it for them on "compassionate grounds". It made, however, one stipulation. The patients' physicians had to promise to keep records of their progress and submit completed reports to the department in the early 1980s

Myth: **The Canadian Government directed that Rene could use Essiac to treat cancer patients subject to the following conditions:**

- **that only medically certified terminal cases should receive treatment.**
- **that records of all patients should be kept and be available for examination at any time.**
- **that she should receive no payment for her work.**

Reality: Extensive research has failed to produce written evidence of any directive from the Canadian government pertaining to this. After presenting her cases at a hearing convened by Dr. J.A. Faulkner, Minister of Health, at Rene's request, sometime in 1934, she was given verbal permission to carry on treating patients, directing that she *"must try and get the doctor's written diagnoses"* but he did not say it was compulsory.

She would continue to work without charge. No mention was made of the Canadian government having any legal right of interest in the written records and the patients did not have to be terminally ill in order to be treated. A lot of them came to have their ulcers treated.

She had written to Dr. Faulkner after having yet another health officer appear on her doorstep with a warrant for her arrest for *"practicing medicine without a license."* She always said she lost count of the number of times over the years she was threatened with arrest and imprisonment for treating patients with the formula.

By her own choice, Rene did not make any charges for the treatment.

"The look of gratitude I saw in their eyes when relief from pain was accomplished, and the hope and cheerfulness that returned when they saw their malignancies reducing, was pay enough for all my efforts."

Rene was a very organised and methodical worker, keeping records as far as the work load allowed. Patients either came to the clinic of their own volition or because their doctors, friends or family wanted them to.

"The look of gratitude I saw in their eyes when there was relief of pain, and the hope and cheerfulness that returned when they saw their malignancies reducing, was pay enough for all my efforts."

Myth: Essiac can be classified as a cure for a number of disorders, including cancer, and should therefore be categorised as a drug.

Reality: Essiac has been shown to have remedial and palliative properties with various diseases, including cancer, and when used in conjunction with conventional therapies such as chemotherapy and radiotherapy, but the recipe is primarily a food supplement which is why it is called a herbal 'tea'. It is not a drug and therefore cannot be classified as such.

During a two-year judicial trial in Hull, Quebec, at which Sheila testified, a company manufacturing a decoction using the same herbs as those in the Essiac recipe was cited for advertising its product as a cure for cancer without applying for a Drug Identification number. The resulting adjudication classified the product as a food, not a drug. One of the defence attorneys presented the court with the following definitions:

Food: A natural substance or combination of bio-organic substances containing nutrients or nutritive products to:
- maintain and support living tissues
- permit the regeneration of living cells
- supply energy for the physiological equilibrium within an organism

Drug: A substance or combination of substances, usually made of synthetic or isolated compounds and matter (other than food) that alters or modifies:

- the physical state
- the psychological state
- the emotional state

Remedy: A substance or combination of substances usually originating from a natural source that can correct the physiological equilibrium within an organism.

Conclusion: Food can be remedial without being a drug.
Essiac can be remedial and is not a drug.

Myth: Rene Caisse tested the formula on 55,000 people.
Reality: Logically and mathematically this must be an exaggeration. These figures relate primarily to the period from 1936 to 1939 when Rene was not only responsible for operating her clinic but also acquiring the herbs and preparing the remedy herself. One woman, working primarily alone and without the sophisticated laboratory and communications equipment we take for granted today, could neither have produced enough herbal tea to treat so many people nor kept so many written records. Anyone who has harvested the herbs and made up the decoction in any quantity knows just how long and how much hard work it takes.

Nevertheless the number of people Rene treated with her formula is impressive by any standards, as are the thousands of signatures collected in her support in 1938.

Myth: There is documented evidence dating from the 1930s showing the complete recovery of thousands of cancer patients who had been certified in writing by their doctors as incurable.
Reality: Records of hundreds of patients with cancer and other serious health conditions were kept by Rene during the 1930s. Some doctors signed written diagnoses but, by 1937, most were reluctant to commit their signatures to such statements.

She testified to the two examining Commissioners who visited the clinic in 1939 to *"between twelve hundred and fifteen hundred* (patients) *in the past three years."*

Myth: **Rene achieved an 80% success rate using the tea.**
Reality: Rene never once made such a claim. Only a limited number of her written records survive, certainly not sufficient to prove such a figure. From the beginning not all the records were kept.

"Sometimes if the patients did not come back we just tore up the cards and threw them away."

Myth: **Rene kept the freely given Native American formula secret because she was self-seeking and arrogant.**
Reality: Let her speak for herself, as she testified under oath to the Commissioners:

"I was afraid that with all the money being spent on radium and X-ray and those sort of things, that it being a simple treatment, they would shelve it without a full enough investigation of its merits. You know how people are sort of inclined to scoff at anything simple and the deeper things interest them much more. I was just afraid that it would not be given a fair test whether it had merit or not. I thought that if I cured enough people, it could not be disputed, and I would be sure that when I handed it over to the medical profession, that it would be made available to the cancer sufferers."

Myth: **All Rene's work was destroyed by the Canadian government after her death.**
Reality: The Canadian government was not involved in any way. Rene's relatives were left to clear her house after her death. They had an auction of her personal effects on the front lawn and one woman bought one of her paintings for $1.50 without knowing what she was buying. No one had the time to go through all the paperwork, no government officials came to claim it and a lot of it was burned one weekend in the back yard.

Myth: **Rene measured the herbs in the original recipe in 'parts by weight'.**
Reality: Rene never measured the herbs in 'parts by weight'.

Some people who have subsequently interpreted the entire recipe in 'parts by weight' have created a completely unbalanced formula, e.g. they have weighed out fifty-two ounces of Burdock root (approximately 3.25lbs) instead of measuring fifty-two ounces in volume (approximately 1.5lbs).

When Rene was making up the decoction she always measured by volume (which is the North American domestic method). Two ounces of the dry herb mix would be measured as two fluid ounces volume in a measuring cup. Many people have interpreted the recipe as two ounces in weight, effectively doubling the strength and more. If Rene knew today that some people were taking nine ounces of more than double strength tea every day (as given in some recommendations), she would be absolutely horrified.

Myth: **Colloidal silver helps preserve Essiac in storage.**
Reality: Please don't. There is absolutely no need to use any kind of preservative in the decoction. If the bottles are sterilised and the formula is made up and stored correctly, it will maintain strength and freshness without any addition. Adding something like colloidal silver could dramatically alter its entire synergy and might be dangerous.

Myth: **While Rene was working with Charles Brusch she added Kelp, Red clover, Blessed thistle and Watercress to her basic four-herb recipe.**
Reality: There is no evidence that Rene added these herbs to the four she was working on. The original recipe given to her in 1922 contained eight herbs which included Red clover and Watercress. Kelp and Blessed thistle were not part of the original recipe. She used the watercress cautiously and selectively.

Myth: **Rene gave her patients a minimum of two fluid ounces of Essiac daily.**
Reality: It was Dr. Brusch who first decided that the daily dose should be two fluid ounces of the tea and it was he who first decided to measure the dry herb mixture by weight rather than volume.

Sheila acted as an emissary between him and Rene Caisse for a short time in 1977. He had begged Rene for enough of the tea to treat one patient. She sent him what she considered to be sufficient for a three months supply of the ready-mixed herbs. In less than one month he had used all of it and was asking for more. Rene asked him, *"Who are you giving it to? Are you giving it to other doctors? What are you doing with it? I sent you enough for three months."*

"No, you didn't", he replied.

Sheila called him on Rene's behalf and explained that Rene used weight for measuring the bulk mix, but just switched over to a measuring cup {volume} when she portioned out the herbs for making the decoction. If she used eight ounces of herbs to eight quarts of water, she used a measuring cup *in volume* of 8 oz. and there's a lot of difference between weight and volume.

He was adamant.

"No, you use weight", he said.

When one of the packages of the herbal mixture was confiscated at the Canada/USA border later in 1977, the American Medical Association warned Dr. Brusch to cease administering the Essiac formula. However he did not lose interest in it and used what he had left in stock on his one remaining American patient.

When Sheila visited him at his clinic in Massachusetts in 1979, he was still confused, insisting on using weight in preference to volume to measure the formula and would not be persuaded to change his method. He received only small amounts of the dried Essiac herbs, first from Rene and later from Mary. His wife made the decoction for him during the 1980s after he had been diagnosed with cancer.

Unfortunately, this weight/volume confusion continues today, resulting in a number of incorrect recipes and dosages being given.

Myth: **You can drink as much of the tea as you like every day with no side effects.**
Reality: When the recipe has been made up at double or triple strength and taken at two or three times Rene's recommenda-

tion, stomach cramps, headaches, rashes and diarrhoea have been noted in some people. These symptoms may also be indicative of Yellow dock having been substituted for the Sheep sorrel.

"No acute toxicity was seen with Essiac in the MSKCC (Memorial Sloan-Kettering Cancer Clinic) tests, although there was said to be a slight weight loss in treated animals. The NCI (U.S. National Cancer Institute), however, claimed to see lethal toxicity at the highest concentrations in Essiac given to animals," Ralph Moss, *Cancer Therapy*, 1992.

Myth: **Essiac contains a high oxalic acid content, causing kidney stones and aggravating stomach ulcers.**
Reality: The formula must be mixed correctly and the decoction diluted as directed, especially for people who have stomach cancer or ulcers. Here lies the paradox. Both Sheep sorrel and Turkey rhubarb root contain oxalic acid which, in concentration, can aggravate stomach ulcers. But Essiac, containing all four herbs in their entirety, has a proven track record as a remedy for all kinds of ulcers. We have absolutely no record either written or spoken of anyone who has been using the tea long-term having contracted either kidney or bladder stones.

Oxalic acid stimulates the peristaltic functions in the body and also helps the sluggish, prolapsed intestines to regain their normal functions. Studies have shown that Oxalic acid causes a rapid reduction in blood coagulation time, making it valuable in treating haemorrhaging.

Oxalic acid, occurring naturally, is always found in combination with sodium, potassium, calcium, iron and manganese in the juices of many plants such as rhubarb, sorrel, oak bark and yellow dock.

Oxalic acid prepared artificially by oxidising sugar and starch with nitric acid is one of the most powerful escharotic poisons known. Acute oxalic acid toxicity in humans is caused by local corrosive action in the gut and by absorption and excretion of the soluble oxalate.

Dr. Edward E. Shook wrote in his *'Advanced Treatise on Herbology'*:

"The same acid in the form of iron oxalate, potassium, sodium or calcium oxalates, as found in rhubarb (stems) and in sorrel leaves, is quite harmless and those herbs are consumed in great quantities by both man and animals. Rhubarb is one of our best laxative and blood purifying herbs... Sheep sorrel has also been used for reducing adipose (excess fatty) tissue, in the treatment of foul and sloughing ulcers and for cancer. Several of our very best therapeutic agents are members of this family; all of them contain iron, each and every one of them contains oxalates from 2-40%."

Myth: You only need the leaves and the stems of the Sheep sorrel plant for use in the formula.

Reality: In a letter to Dr. Stock at Memorial Sloan-Kettering Center in 1974, Rene stated that as a result of her early experiments on mice inoculated with human cancer, her conclusion was *"the herb that will destroy a cancer (a malignant growth) is Sorrel, the dog-eared Sheep sorrel sometimes called Sourgrass. The entire plant must be used, picked in the Spring before the seeds form, then dried and powdered."*

In a subsequent letter to Dr. Stock, dated August 1975, she writes, *"the material I sent was grown and prepared for grinding into powder (leaves, stems and roots) and boiled. Let stand overnight (12 hours) then poured off into sterile bottles. Do not strain through cheese cloth or anything else."*

Myth: You can substitute the Turkey rhubarb root using the domestic rhubarb root at double strength.

Reality: The recipe uses one ounce of rhubarb root to every sixteen ounces of Sheep sorrel, regardless of which rhubarb is available. Using domestic rhubarb at double strength might significantly increase the oxalic acid level and will introduce the hormonal effect of glycoside rhaponticin which should be used with caution.

Myth: It is important that all the herbal residue be strained out of the tea before using.

Reality: Essiac needs only be strained through a standard kitchen sieve before bottling. Rene wrote in her letter of August 4th 1975 to Dr. Stock that *"to strain it through cheese cloth destroys it."*

All bottles of correctly prepared tea have a residue of the herbs at the bottom. You can either shake it up and drink it as part of the tea or you can pour off the clear liquid as you use it. It's entirely a question of taste and we have no evidence of either method being preferable.

Myth: **There is no need to powder the Sheep sorrel before using it in the decoction.**
Reality: Rene was quite specific about this. She powdered the Sheep sorrel as a result of her early experiments with the remedy. It must be remembered that she paid particular attention to the herb, often injecting it separately, again as a result of the experiments on the tumours in mice. Using the chopped herb upsets the entire balance of the formula. Yes, it may make the initial decoction less murky before it settles, but it also means that the Sheep sorrel will be less concentrated in the tea.

Myth: **If you mix the herbs with good intention, variations in proportion don't matter.**
Reality: No one can fault good intention but, without the sound backing of meticulous research and experience, good intention can just as easily mix up an ineffective or possibly dangerous variation in the proportion of the herbs.

For example, a concentration of Turkey rhubarb root could irritate the intestines and cause abdominal cramping. Burdock root in concentration could overly stimulate the uterus and *"may precipitate a symptomatic crisis in severely toxic conditions or where eliminatory channels are deficient"*. – Simon Mills, 1994

Good intention can never be a substitute for knowledge and experience, especially when someone else's life and wellbeing are at stake. A terminal diagnosis is a terminal diagnosis and deserves the very best of all treatment, both in conventional and alternative therapies.

If you don't agree, wait until the day comes when you are sitting in the chair opposite the doctor and he is looking everywhere but directly at your face, because he doesn't know how to tell you that he has run out of ideas. When the void opens at your feet and making up a bottle of this herbal tea might be the only hope you have left, you will want it to be made of the very best herbs in correct proportion to give you the best possible chance of quality and quantity of life.

Myth: **The herbs should only be mixed according to the phases of the moon.**
Reality: This is entirely a matter of personal belief and no one has the right to impose their theories on any one else. What might be correct according to one system of belief may directly belie another. Diseases have a more impartial view; they happily affect anyone, regardless of whatever godhead.

If your belief system dictates that the herbs must only be harvested and mixed at a certain point in the cycle of the moon, then please follow that. If the weather, family and work obligations or urgency connected with the gravity of a diagnosis mean that you can only harvest the herbs or make the tea at whatever time is available, please be assured that the herbs will be just as potent for you.

Myth: **If you don't like the taste, it's OK to wash Essiac down with an alcoholic drink.**
Reality: You stand a very good chance of vomiting if you do. It appears that Essiac does not mix gladly with alcohol, especially spirits. The body recognises alcohol as a poison and the tea seems to agree. We have had several reports where people have refused to carry on taking the tea because they vomited very soon after drinking it alongside their customary alcoholic night-cap.

However this does not mean that you cannot enjoy a glass of wine with a meal or a drop of any other favourite tipple at some other time of the day, if you absolutely must.

Myth: **It's not necessary to steep the herbs for ten to twelve hours.**

Reality: The roots and the bark need time to fully absorb the water in order to release their medicinal properties. The old native medicine man, who was the originator of the formula, boiled and steeped the herbs, Rene did the same. Like she said, *"If it works, don't change it."*

Myth: The four herbs work equally well in tincture and capsule form.
Reality: Having tried both, we can only say that we choose not to use either of them.

In capsule form the herbs are uncooked, they have not been soaked or steeped to extract the full medicinal properties. They have also been ground down to a very fine powder. Anyone who has ever ground roots or herbs knows that you have to monitor the process very carefully so as not to subject the herbs to the excessive heat engendered by the mechanical grinding process. The finer the powder, the longer the herbs are in the machine and the hotter they get. The capsule contains the dried herbs in concentrated form and can present an absorption problem for some people with digestive disorders.

Tinctures can be made by combining powdered or thoroughly crushed herbs with alcohol diluted with water to make a 50% solution. This mixture is shaken and allowed to stand in a warm place for two weeks, shaken and stirred daily. The resulting liquid is strained off from the herbal residue, taking care to squeeze out as much of the extract as possible. The tincture is kept in a dark bottle and administered by dropper in amounts averaging from one to thirty drops, depending on the herb used. Some tinctures on the market are sold in plastic bottles, which is definitely not a good idea.

> *The old native medicine man, who was the originator of the formula, boiled and steeped the herbs, Rene did the same.*

Rene never considered using the herbs in tincture form as she believed that the traditional boiling method was by far the best method, and the cheapest.

The old medicine man didn't do it; she didn't do it.

Chapter Nine

The Evidence
– What they Said Then

Many people have played a part in the history of Essiac – including doctors, commissioners, investigators, scientific researchers and, of course, the patients themselves.

This chapter identifies the principal characters, examining their contribution to Essiac as we know it today. It also includes important personal testimonies about Essiac from patients, both past and present.

The Principal Characters

Dr. R.O. Fisher:

He was one of the doctors in Toronto with whom Rene was working as a nurse before she began to use the herbs. He supervised her while she was treating her aunt with the tea and was instrumental in helping her to experiment with and to refine the recipe, making it more effective.

Dr. J.A. McInnes:

He was very supportive of Rene's work and introduced her to Dr. Banting. He was a frequent visitor to the Bracebridge Clinic and occasionally helped by examining some of her patients.

Dr. Benjamin Leslie Guyatt:

He met Rene in 1936 and was responsible for getting the

Chicago study underway. He was very impressed with her work and often visited the Bracebridge clinic to examine and observe the patients. Rene invited him to be an observer at the Sub-Committee hearing in Bracebridge in February 1939. He was the only medical doctor who was willing to testify on her behalf at the July hearing in Toronto.

Dr. Emma Carson:

She was a retired physician who came from California to visit the clinic in Bracebridge in the summer of 1937. Originally intending to visit for a day, she stayed for a month, keeping meticulous daily notes and became the only doctor to provide a detailed account of how Rene worked to maintain the clinic. She interviewed several hundred patients, many of whom declared themselves returned to normal health.

"*As I seriously and compassionately surveyed that extraordinary assembly of afflicted people and visually compared them with the most prominent and distinguished clinics I have ever witnessed either in this (USA) or foreign countries, I vividly realised that I had never before seen or been in any manner associated with such a remarkably cheerful and sympathetic clinic, regardless of size, location or number of persons; or attended a more peaceful, sympathetic clinic anywhere.*"

Dr. Richard Leonardo:

A coroner from Rochester, NY, who was a cancer specialist and wrote several books on the subject. He came into the Bracebridge Clinic out of curiosity while he was holidaying in Muskoka. At first he was very sceptical but after a day and a half observing the patients he was definitely impressed. Three years later he wrote a letter to the Cancer Commission refuting his earlier statements saying that he did not believe that Essiac had actually helped the patients.

Jim Kennedy:

He was a businessman from Buffalo, NY, who offered one million dollars cash to Rene in 1937, plus access to a new building for the clinic. Those patients who did not have the means would be treated there without charge. The offer was made in November 1937 followed by a personal letter to Rene from Jim Kennedy in February 1938, making the offer conditional on the Private Members Bill being passed in Parliament the following March. The Bill failed and nothing more came of the offer.

Ralph Daigh:
He was the vice-president and editorial director of Fawcett Publications in New York and was responsible for introducing Rene to Dr. Brusch.

Dr Charles Brusch:
He was a medical doctor who was treating his patients with vitamin and mineral supplements as early as the 1950s.

Rene cooperated with him briefly from May 1959 until June 1960, working with him at The Brusch Medical Centre in Cambridge, Massachusetts, using Essiac in a trial involving eight human subjects and a number of mice injected with human carcinoma. The animal trials were the most immediately successful and caught the attention of the researchers at the Memorial Sloan Kettering Institute in New York. When Rene refused to give them the formula because they would not guarantee her any recognition for the work she had done, they took measures to ensure that the trials would be closed down by cutting off the supply of research material and resources.

There is no record of any further correspondence between Rene and Dr Brusch until a letter headed 'Brusch Medical Center' and dated September 21st 1976.

"Dear Rene,
I am sorry if seemingly I have failed to communicate with you. I say seemingly purposely because I felt quite positive I had answered all the letters I received from you.

As you know, I am still interested in your project and wish you the best of success always. In addition, I am ready to cooperate with you in any way I can. I do have a few cases here who might be interested in cooperating also. Perhaps I am a little out of touch with present conditions – but do communicate with me and let me know specifically in what way you would like me to assist you.

Best of luck always, Rene. I shall look forward to hearing from you.

Sincerely,

Charles A. Brusch, MD.*"*

In 1977 he requested some of the ready mixed herbs to treat a few Canadian patients who had been referred to him by Rene after she had been cautioned about supplying Essiac to patients personally. The records of only one American patient were retained. Dr. Brusch acted as Rene's advisor during the negotiations with the Resperin Corporation and, together with Doctor Rynard, witnessed the agreement signed on October 26th 1977. There is no evidence to suggest or to prove that Rene ever gave him the recipe. What evidence there is from private correspondence implies that she did not. Equally there is no evidence to prove that he ever entered into any form of a legal partnership with Rene during her lifetime, although mention was made in a letter dated February 21 1980 from Resperin's lawyers to Dr Brusch denying his request for royalties, that David Fingard had previously referred to his 'partnership' with Rene. In a letter to Mary McPherson dated January 28th 1986, Dr. Brusch refers to a document obtained when he brought suit against Resperin which states that *"Rene and I had an oral agreement"*.

Dr Chester Stock:

As the Vice-President for Academic Affairs, Memorial Sloan-Kettering Cancer Center, he corresponded with Rene for three years during the early 1970s while he was involved in carrying out trials on mice inoculated with animal carcinoma, using a decoction of the Sheep sorrel rather than all four herbs. It is evident from the tone of her letters that Rene became increasingly mistrustful of the nature of the trials and how they were being conducted. The investigation was halted in 1976.

Eleanor Sniderman:

She was a well-known and highly respected Toronto businesswoman who came to Bracebridge to meet Rene in 1977 after the *Homemakers* magazine article was published. Eventually she persuaded the Lieutenant-Governor to accept a sealed envelope from Rene containing the details of the formula.

The Hon. Pauline McGibbon:

She was the Lieutenant-Governor of the Province of Ontario who accepted the sealed envelope from Rene in August 1977 and deposited it in her private vault. She personally returned it to Rene when the contract was being signed with the Resperin Corporation.

Dr. David Walde:

He was the oncologist from Sault St. Marie, Ontario, who was introduced to the magazine article by his own patients. In July 1977, he persuaded Rene to allow him sufficient supplies of the dried herbs to begin oral treatment on twenty volunteer patients to whom no other conventional treatment could be offered.

Dr. John Barker:

He was a doctor from Port Credit, west of Toronto, who was persuaded to treat the Canadians who were turned away from the Brusch Clinic by the American Medical Association in 1977. He collected his first limited supply of the liquid formula from Rene at the end of July and began treating fifteen patients.

{Both the Walde and Barker trials lasted only three months and were terminated as inconclusive.}

David Fingard:

An elderly retired chemist, he was the Head of the Resperin Corporation, a small Toronto-based drug company which had been responsible for a single product based on creosote and phenol for treating asthma. The production was closed down by the Health Department in 1970. The company was scouting for another product and became interested in Rene's work as a result of the *Homemakers* article. David Fingard promised to set up clinical trials in return for having the exclusive right to market the formula.

After Rene signed the formal agreement with the company in October 1977, Canadian doctors were invited to apply to Resperin for supplies of Essiac to treat specific patients. Initially over a hundred patients were treated with the formula but an increasing lack of interest on the part of the doctors involved meant that the results of the treatment were never fully reported. Many of the report forms were never returned and the company was reported as being disappointed in the response to the trials.

Resperin had the name 'Essiac' officially registered as a trademark on August 1st 1980, registration number 249752. The directors transferred the Corporation's rights to their formula and name to another company in Campbelltown, New Brunswick, in 1991.

Stephen Roman:

He was a wealthy man who reportedly invested a quarter of a million dollars with the Resperin Corporation to fund the trials to test the formula.

Dr Matthew Dymond:

A doctor and former Minister of Health for Ontario, he was put in charge of making up the decoction by the Resperin Corporation after Rene had signed over the formula. He had arranged to visit Rene at her home so that she could take him step by step through the process of making Essiac, but she broke her hip and was admitted to hospital the day before they were due to meet. She was never well enough to see him again and it was left to Mary McPherson to teach him how to prepare the formula until he felt sufficiently confident in handling the work himself.

The Witnesses

What They Said Then

At the Sub-Committee hearing, Bracebridge Clinic, Friday and Saturday, February 3rd and 4th 1939.
Appearances: Dr. R.C. Wallace, Dr. T.H. Callahan.
          Official Reporter Mr R. Brydie

Former patients of Rene Caisse were called to testify at the court hearing.

Mrs M.N, questioned by:
Commissioner Wallace:

Q This is being taken down so that the other members of the Commission may know about it. You will speak so that the gentleman here can hear well.

A Well, ask me any questions and I am prepared to answer them.

Q You had an examination by Dr. Shannon in St. Michael's Hospital or by some other doctor?

A Dr. Bateman.

Q Dr. Shannon probably read the plates?

A He took the X-ray plates.

Q That was this year?

A That was in March I think.

Q In March of 1938?

A Yes.

Q X-ray plates were taken...

A Yes.

Q ...by Dr.Bateman in March?
A I think it was in March.

Commissioner Callahan:
Q 1938?
A Yes, and I came up here in May. It was March or April I had them, and I came up here in May for the first treatment.

Commissioner Wallace:
Q The reference to the plates by Dr. Shannon is April 4th?
A About that time.
   Exhibit No.44: Clinic card, Mrs F.M.N, May 10th 1938
   Exhibit No.45: Diagnosis re: Mrs F.M.N, April 4th 1938
Q You took no treatment at that time?
A No.
Q What did Dr. Bateman advise you should do?
A He advised getting the x-ray, and after that he said that if they did operate they would open the bowel out at the side, and my husband said he would not have that.
Q You refused the operation?
A Yes. At that time I was sitting with a hot water bottle on night and day. I just felt I was going to die; I did not have any ambition to do anything.
Q You had had trouble for a long time?
A Yes but Dr. Bateman did not think it was serious until I went up to him in April, and he said he thought before it was sacs on the bowel. I had appendicitis some years ago, and I had come in several times, and he...

Commissioner Callahan:
Q Did he operate upon you at that time?
A No, I was very young when I had the operation. Then Mr N brought me here, and after the third treatment I began to get better.
Q You came up here when?
A In May 1938. At that time I had a woman doing my work, and now I can do it myself.

Commissioner Wallace:

Q How many treatments have you had?

A I have had about 23.

Q Are you taking them regularly Mrs N?

A Once a week. I have diabetes too. I take insulin twice a day, but Miss Caisse has dried up the sugar. I have not had it as bad as I had when I had it first.

Q You took insulin?

A Yes. I skip it once a day very often now that I am getting so much better. I have had that for 12 years.

Commissioner Callahan:

Q You have taken insulin for that long?

A No, sir. I have taken insulin for about 6 years.

Commissioner Wallace:

Q What is your condition now?

A It is very much better. I go out and just do what I like, and I have not felt so well for 15 years as I do now.

Q You propose to continue the treatment for some time?

A Yes, as long as Miss Caisse keeps open I come to her. I think she has done wonderful work. If she did not do any more than she has done for me, it is miraculous. You would not know me today. When I went into a store the other day the man nearly dropped dead; he thought I would be buried.

Q You have gained weight?

A No, I have not gained weight; I have just lost a little. I weighed 154 when I came up here first, and I am down to 148 now.

Commissioner Callahan:

Q You have not lost much weight?

A No, but I think it is due to doing my own work, and hustling around. I sat around quite a lot, and was not able to. I had the pain here (indicating) and I just held my side, and that is all I could do. At night I would just toss around, and would not get any sleep.

Commissioner Wallace:

Q You have no pain at all?

A I have some pain yet; it has an uncomfortable feeling there, but it is not anything as bad as it was. You can imagine that, when I am doing my own work myself. I go around and out around every day, and I do my own work. I was just discouraged and I had just given up. I did not expect to be living today. I went in to have a new plate made by the dentist, and I thought I would be ordering a coffin instead of a plate.

Commissioner Callahan:

Q You have taken how many treatments?

A Twenty-three.

Commissioner Wallace:

Q It is given on the card as twenty-four.

A I keep track of them.

Q Did they affect you in any way?

A Well, I had a reaction last Saturday.

Q Of what kind?

A Chills and fever.

Q Chills and fever?

A I just felt as though I was getting a cold, and I laid down and slept for three hours, and when I got up it was all right.

Q Was that during the same day?

A Yes, that Saturday. I got home and had my dinner, and I got chilly. I thought I was getting a cold because I got into the cold car, but it was a reaction all right. I have had two of them. Miss Caisse is doing wonderful work.

Commissioner Wallace:

That is all.

*   *   *   *   *

Mrs E.F., questioned by:
Commissioner Wallace:

We are taking a record so that other members of this Commission will get the information as well, and in order to do that, we ask that you take an affirmation that what you say is true.

A Very well.

Q And if could you speak so that you can be heard by this gentleman, the reporter, we will appreciate that.

A Yes.

...Whereupon the witness sworn.

Commissioner Callahan:

Q You know, you do not need to mind this?

A No.

Q You do not feel a bit nervous about this?

A No, not in a way.

Q Do not be, because we want to hear about these things. It is very interesting and we want to hear it.

A Do you just want me to tell my story?

Commissioner Wallace:

I think we might ask questions a little bit, because you have a very long story, I believe.

A Yes.

Q Did Dr. Greig give you any letter or make any statement when he examined you before you began taking treatments here?

A No, he did not. He told me when I went that I was supposed to go back to him again, but the examination hurt me so much, and I bled so badly after the examination, that I...

Commissioner Callahan:

Q You mean the vaginal examination?

A Yes. I just came back to Miss Caisse and begged her to give me the treatment, and she did, and after I had taken them a short time this all cleared up.

Q The bleeding?

A Yes, and there was a discharge mixed with pus as well before that. That is what aroused my suspicion in the beginning was this terrible discharge. I would have to change my clothing almost every day. So I came to Dr. Greig and he examined me. Of course, Dr. Greig is not my own doctor, but my own doctor was away and I went to Dr. Greig.

Commissioner Wallace:

Q Was your doctor Dr. Bastedo?

A Yes.

Q You were attending him before that time?

A Yes.

Q In 1929 he operated upon you?

A Yes, and they always told me that those growths were not cancerous growths, but the last time when I had radium they said that they were very suspicious, you see, but yet they never said it was cancer. After the operation they returned, you see.

Q How long did you take radium treatments?

A 36 hours. They gave me one treatment of 36 hours.

Q That was in 1931, was it?

A Yes.

Q In the Toronto General Hospital?

A No sir, in the Grace Hospital.

Q There was no radium treatment on the Toronto General Hospital?

A No, I was under Dr. Wales at that time.

Q So you have had neither radium treatment nor an operation since 1931?

A No, I have not had anything like that since then.

Q Since 1931?

A No.

Q You had an examination in 1937?

A Yes.

Q By Dr. Greig?

A Yes.

Q And you took treatment in May 1937?

A Yes.

Q That is the picture.

A Yes.

Q Tell us about the situation since that time, since you began to take treatments.

A Well, since then I have just greatly gained in health, and there is not any discharge at the present time. I have a family of nine, and there are nine of us in the house, and I do all my own work, and make my own beds. I make my own bread, and butter, and do my own washing and cleaning, etc., all the time, and in the past since before Christmas I came to Miss Caisse, and I gained four pounds since then.

Q You came to Miss Caisse?

A I have not been having my treatments since before Christmas.

Q I understand you now. You had your treatments much earlier?

A Sure. I have been taking treatments since 1937.

Q Continuously except in the spring?

A Yes, except when the Clinic would not be open, but since before Christmas I have not been able to yet because my husband was thrown off a truck and nearly had his back broken, and since then I have not been having my treatment, but still I have been gaining in weight. I really feel that I owe my life to Miss Caisse.

Q You are feeling quite well now?

A Yes, quite well.

Q In every way?

A Yes.

Q How much weight have you gained altogether since you began to take the treatment, do you think?

A At first I went down. When I first started the treatment the reaction was very severe, and I went down. I weigh 148 today, and I weighed 102, when I started.

Q How did the treatment affect you?

A They make me hot and cold, and that is about all there is to it, that I can say. Of course it makes the parts sore, you know. I always had it in the muscular part of the limb.

Q Do you perspire?

A No, I do not think I ever did.

Q Would you permit me to examine you if the nurse prepares you?

A Well, I suppose you can.

Q You have no objection to my examining you?

A No, if you don't hurt me too badly.

Q I do not think I will.

A I have had so many examinations that I am kind of tired.

Commissioner Callahan:
Well, I will see if I can arrange for you to be prepared.
Exhibit No. 3: Clinic card re. Mrs J.C.F., May 2nd, 1937.

Later insert:
Commissioner Callahan:
I might say here, Commissioner Wallace, that in Mrs. F's case, I have just finished the vaginal examination. On examination of the cervix-uteri, this appeared to be free of any growth or ulceration. I made this examination with a bi-valve speculum, and I found the cervix to be absolutely normal. I also made a bi-manual examination and found the uterus to be atrophied. There was no haemorrhage.

The witness retired.

*　　*　　*　　*　　*

Mr S. H, questioned by:
Commissioner Wallace:
Q You are Mr S.H. of Huntsville, Ontario?
A Yes.

Commissioner Wallace:
Exhibit No. 24: Diagnosis by two physicians re Mr. S. H., March 27, 1937.
Exhibit No. 25: Clinic card, re Mr. S. H.

Commissioner Wallace:
Q You went into the Orillia Hospital for X-rays?
A Yes. That is about two years ago...a year ago. In 1937, in March.
Q In March, 1937?
A I think it was March.

Q And you had a plate taken at that time?

A I had five or six taken.

Q Five or six plates. Was a diagnosis made of you there, or did they tell you what was the matter?

A Yes.

Q What did they say?

A They said I had a very serious trouble; I had a growth in between my two stomachs, ... in between my two stomachs they said there was a diseased growth. I have a little story if you are ready.

Commissioner Wallace:
You just go right ahead but do it slowly.

The Witness:
I said how would I get it out of there if I did not have an operation, and he said I would have to have an operation, and, "you cannot get it out of there unless you have an operation" I thought all the time I would come and see Miss Caisse though. He said "You can go home now, and talk this over with your boys, and if they decide on having an operation, you come back, and I will send the plates to Toronto to my uncle, and he will operate on you."

I came home, and I came to Miss Caisse, and I told her about it, and she said, "Who is your doctor?" and I said, "I have practically really no doctor, but I went to Dr. Evans and he thought it was indigestion I had, and he gave me a bottle of something, and I took a few doses of it, and it didn't do any good". Miss Caisse said, "You are very wise not to have an operation." I said, "Do you think I am?" She said, "Yes, I know it." I said, "Do you think you can do me good?" and she said "Yes, I can." I said, "I am very pleased to hear it. You can give me treatments and I will come and take them". I did, and I took about eleven, and on the following 14th of August, I felt it leave my stomach and it went right out of me. Everything before that that I passed was as thin as water, and I felt this go down and on and out of me. I was very foolish in not catching it. It seemed to be about 4 inches long and about three-quarters of an inch in diameter.

Q That is the cancer?

A Well, it was the growth that was there .... whatever it was. It might have been a cancer; I do not know anything about it.

Q You felt this thing go on through?

A I certainly did. It went through me and out of me. I could feel it about four inches long and about three-quarters of an inch in size. After that I could eat anything I liked. I felt so good I felt hungry, and I felt so good, I could just eat what I wanted to eat. Now I can eat anything but the real sour things, such as pickles and that, which really go against me. It seems as though they will not digest properly and will give me pain. I can eat anything else, especially lots of meat, good fat bacon and pork, and I can eat that all along.

Q How long did you continue the treatment?

A Well, I took eleven, and this left me, and I took on and off from that. I took about a month regular every week and since that I have only taken them in about three weeks, and, in the most, two months. Last, I think, I was down here between the 1st and the 4th – along there – and I have not been here since the last of November.

Commissioner Callahan:

Q Before you took these treatments, were you eating very well?

A No.

Q If you ate a full meal what would happen?

A Well, it would lay in my stomach and I would vomit it out.

Q Did that happen very often?

A Well, I guess about 100 times or more.

Q Did you lose weight?

A Yes. I dropped 22 pounds in about two weeks.

Q Have you gained it back?

A Yes, I have gained it back now. I was hardly normal. I am within 2 or 3 pounds of being normal now.

Q You have weighed up to 157?

A Yes, I have weighed up to 170 and 165, along there, and then 150 and 155 pounds, and sometimes it would drop to about 150, but I certainly believe if I had not come here I would have been dead long before this.

Q Did you take other treatment...

A No.

Q ...of any kind?

A No. She did wonderful work for me.

Q Do you feel quite well in every way?

A Yes, I feel fine.

Q Do you do any work?

A Yes.

Q What is your occupation?

A Well, now I do any job I get a chance to.

Q You live in Huntsville in town?

A Not in town; I have a home out of town, but I can work a long day now.

Q Yes, I see. Thank you very much. You have not far to go today?

A No.

Q That is all.

The witness retired.

* * * * *

In addition to these verbatim testimonies from witnesses to the Commission, records from Rene's Bracebridge Clinic (which we have seen) contain many accounts from individual patients testifying to the benefits they received from Essiac in the 1930s.

This one is a perfect example of 'doctors in denial':
MRS T DOUGLAS – Age 43
Copy of pathological report – Public Health Laboratories, Division of Pathology, Department of Health, Ontario.

Douglas, Mrs T   Aug 5th, 1938   T-5214-38

Dr. A L Hoare, Markham, Ontario

Diagnosis: Carcinoma of the cervix

Gross specimen: Consists of a number of irregular small fragments of granular material from the cervix.

Microscopic report: Sections of the tissue show it to be composed largely of fibrous connective tissue which is being infiltrated with great masses of atypical epithelial cells which appear to be arising from squamous epithelium. However, these cells are very poorly differentiated and very malignant, but radiosensitive.

J.A.Ansley, Pathologist

Mrs Douglas had her first treatment at the clinic on August 12th, 1938. She boarded in Bracebridge for six weeks.

"I was an invalid that summer, unable to eat and down to 117 pounds in weight. I went (to Bracebridge) on a bed made in the back of the car, on a mattress with a feather tick folded on it, and I could stand no jolting of the car. As I lay in my bed, I could see the clinic on the hill and it reminded me of the Cross on the Hill of Calvary. It was the only ray of hope I had in the whole world."

On September 24th Rene Caisse recorded: "Patient starting to slough off pieces of growth; feeling and looking very well."

Patient stated, "In six weeks, I had gained 17 pounds, improved my appetite and was able to sleep."

Eight weeks after the first treatment, Mrs Douglas "passed a growth about the size of a baseball but there was much more material that came away outside of that."

December 1938 – patient very well and is very hopeful of a complete cure.

Copy of a letter written to Miss Caisse by Mrs Douglas, Highland Creek, Ontario, December 9th, 1938.

"Miss Rene Caisse
Bracebridge, Ontario.

"Dear Miss Caisse,
"In reviewing the history of my illness, I wish to state that I have not felt well since my boy was born sixteen years ago, but more particularly during the past twelve years after having had a fall in a fire. I have had medical attention by the best of family physicians during all that time but not one of these doctors was able to diagnose the source of my illness nor would they recommend specialists at my request, as they felt they were fully confident of their ability to terminate my suffering.

"During the past three years, I suffered untold agony with pains in my back for which doctors gave me opiates and nerve tonic, even though I had informed the doctors that I was functioning irregularly, similar to a state of menopause, at the early age of forty.

"On March 16th, 1938, I experienced a most unnatural flow which continued from that date right through until October 1938, at which time I noticed a considerable cessation of my condition.

"My doctor was attending me regularly. On June 27th, 1938, when he saw that I failed to respond to his treatment, he admitted that my condition needed hospitalisation. My husband took me to Dr. Frawley, chief gynaecologist of St. Michael's Hospital, and he instantly diagnosed my case as cancer of the cervix and uterus, caused he thought by a chronic condition of unhealed lacerations at childbirth. Dr. Frawley advised hospitalisation for removal of tissue for verification of his diagnosis by the Pathological Department of Health but, as I was not well enough at the time to take ether, I went to my sister's (at Markham) for a rest. She took me to her doctor's office where he removed tissue from the affected parts which he took to the pathological department himself. The report came back that the tissues had shown malignant cancer.

"The doctor advised hospitalisation, radium and deep X-ray treatment. He advised that I had only twenty per cent chance of a cure and that, if I didn't take radium, my chances to live would be limited to approximately four years. Three of my friends, neighbour women, had had similar treatment and died within three years. They told me they were dying a death of fiery internal furnace. So, knowing of their untimely deaths and awful agony, I was determined to die comfortably if needs be by the inroads of cancerous growths rather than take radium and die as well in agony.

"I heard of the Rene Caisse Cancer Clinic and started my treatments there in August 1938. I was an invalid, unable to do my own housework or eat, weighing 117 pounds and becoming weaker every day. But today, December 9th, thank God, I weigh 130 pounds, I eat three full-course meals a day, do my own housework as well as nurse my daughter, recently operated on for appendicitis. I have not had time to become wholly well, but I state definitely that I feel better and stronger since taking this treatment than during the past twelve years. When my doctor saw me last week, he was astounded at my vigorous appearance and radiant health. When I told him that your Caisse cancer treatment had performed the miracle, he immediately defended himself and Dr. Frawley by stating that I evidently did not have cancer at all, as my case must have been diagnosed incorrectly. It appeared to me that he said this only to discredit the benefits of your cancer treatments. But, what he does not know is that the pathological department definitely diagnosed the tissue taken from my cervix or uterus as malignant cancer and sent the result to another doctor.

"I will subject myself to any medical examination that you may recommend in order to prove that your treatment is beneficial to suffering humanity who are deprived of its benefits by antagonistic doctors who are doing all in their power to discredit the merits of your cancer treatment.

"Yours truly,
(signed) Mrs T Douglas."

"I will subject myself to any medical examination that you may recommend in order to prove that your treatment is beneficial to suffering humanity who are deprived of its benefits by antagonistic doctors who are doing all in their power to discredit the merits of your cancer treatment.

When Mrs Douglas testified at the Cancer Commission hearing, she was asked by the Chairman if there had been a subsequent biopsy. She replied that she had gone to be examined by Dr. S. Cosbie at the Toronto General Hospital just one week earlier.

He had told her: "It doesn't look like there is much wrong with you."

She replied: "I only submitted to this examination to console my husband that I was improving."

Dr. Cosbie decided that a scraping wasn't necessary at that time. Patient's weight was back up to 131 pounds when she was examined.

Chapter Ten

What They Say Now

*T*he Essiac formula did not die with Rene in 1978. Ever-increasing numbers of people are discovering and using it. They continue to bear witness to Essiac's remarkable healing qualities. Here is a selection from the many testimonies we have been given:

Mr A.M., Canada, March 1991 – Age 67
December 28th 1987: Lung cancer diagnosed. " I was spitting up blood and knew myself it was likely cancer in March or April of 1987 but was not diagnosed until December. They kept saying if there was something there, they weren't finding it." Initially treated with radiation and a form of chemotherapy at the Falk Clinic in Toronto. "I was only given six months to a year, as of January 1988, to live."

March 1988: Mr M started taking Essiac and immediately felt a sense of wellbeing. He experienced a beneficial change in his eating and elimination habits and had no side effects while taking the tea.

March 14th 1991: "I am feeling very good as of now. I must give Essiac most of the credit for my recovery,"

Autumn, 1992: Mrs M was sent a questionnaire by the Ontario Cancer Institute requesting details of her husband's death! She replied "....He is feeling fine and I feel he is free of the cancer. I feel that Essiac should be given a chance to help every patient, but before treatment is begun, not when given up on and one foot in the grave."

I feel that Essiac should be given a chance to help every patient, but before treatment is begun, not when (he/she is) given up on and (with) one foot in the grave."

May 16th 1995: Mr M continuing to take Essiac and reported that he felt it had built up his immune system and appetite.

August 1997: Still taking Essiac and still very well.

June 1998: Continues to progress. Spent the previous winter refurbishing a house in Toronto.

Mr E.K. Canada, May 1994 – Age 68

May 1993: Malignant tumour in the prostate diagnosed. "As soon as I discovered I had cancer, I started drinking four quarts of carrot juice daily plus raw vegetables and fruit, so I felt my body was detoxified when I started the tea."

August 12th 1993: "They removed my testicles and I was very sick with a lot of pain. I was given shots of morphine."

A course of hormone therapy was recommended (anti-oestrogen Flutamide) but Mr K was unable to tolerate it. There was no improvement in his condition since the tumour had not been removed. "I was told in these words 'the horse is already out of the barn'. The doctor was only trying to prolong my life."

August 16th 1993: "I started taking Essiac (2 fluid ounces daily) and couldn't believe how much better I felt about twelve days later."

September 19th 1993: "I had my last bout with pain. I was able to tolerate the pain with 222s" (strong aspirin tablets).

October 7th 1993: "My PSA (prostate specific antigen) level was 3·0 and it had been 400 on August 4th 1993. Each day I continued to feel so much better ... I was amazed."

November 12th 1993: "I started excreting what looked like a cottage-cheese substance through my penis. This lasted about two weeks."

April 7th 1994: "I was told that I was in good health and that my prostate was normal. My PSA level was ·02 – EXCELLENT! My urologist left the room and never said another

My urologist left the room and never said another word, but our family physician told my wife he got a report from the urologist telling him he was "amazed".

word, but our family physician told my wife he got a report from the urologist telling him he was "amazed". My wife told our family physician that we chose alternative medicine because we knew I could not live for too long with a malignant tumour in my prostate. He said, 'Whatever you have done, continue ... it's a miracle.' My wife and I will always keep the torch burning for Essiac. It's a crime people are dying of cancer when there are cures."

G. O'Shea, UK, June 1998.

"In the summer of 1995 we were living in Spain. During a severe drought lasting around three months, the local water company allowed sea water to flow through our water pipes which we now believe set up a very toxic reaction, causing at least twelve people that I know of to go down with cancer at the same time. Most of us were diagnosed in early 1996.

"After my diagnosis I went into shock. Sadly my local doctor was of no help. After a hysterectomy to remove a 10cm tumour from one of my ovaries, I underwent my first course of chemotherapy which made me feel very ill. I had lost two stones in weight and looked like something out of a concentration camp. I found eating very difficult, I kept passing out and my husband had to lift me in and out of the bath because I was so weak. I am normally such an optimistic person with a great love of life but at that time I didn't think that I was ever going to recover which was so unlike me. I was only forty-six years old.

"I had about fifteen months remission after finishing the chemotherapy. We were back in Spain and I had only just got my life back into some sort of order when the results of my latest C.A. 125 blood test showed that the cancer cells were active again. Although we were devastated by the news, I was determined to be more positive this time. A couple of mornings later I remember saying a little prayer to the angels I had always believed had protected and guided me throughout my life. That same afternoon I answered a knock on the door to find a friend standing there with a leaflet in her hand. It was all about Essiac. I immediately ordered a supply which I have been taking ever since.

"I came back to England in January of this year to start a second course of chemotherapy, still taking the tea. Because it had been almost four months since the secondary cells had been found, my oncologist was convinced that I would have a large tumour or at least several small ones. I had been taking Essiac for about two months. The CT scan returned clear, I believe thanks to Essiac, a healthier diet and an even more positive attitude. My oncologist was very surprised but still put me on to a second six months of chemotherapy because of the active cells.

"The one thing that I have found from all this is that the hospitals continually tell me that I have no hope while all the alternative and complementary practitioners I have come into contact with during these last few months have been so positive. Although I must say that the doctors have been very surprised at how well I have tolerated this second course of chemotherapy and how fit and healthy I have stayed throughout the full six months.

"A lot of other cancer patients I know are now taking Essiac and all of them are doing very well. I've even got my brother to take it for his diabetes. He agreed to take it for a few weeks just to please me and not only did he feel much better but he told me that a small lump he had noticed on his leg for about five months had started to tingle before it gradually disappeared. He wouldn't be without his Essiac now.

"I have noticed a definite difference between those people I know with ovarian cancer who are either taking the tea or using some kind of alternative treatment and those who are not. It's no good just being positive about the cancer and relying on the conventional treatment. You've got to back it up with other therapies like keeping to a special diet or taking the tea. It's important to me how I feel when I am ill and I need to feel well in order to fight back."

S. Champney, UK, May 1998

"I was diagnosed with stage three ovarian cancer following surgery in August 1996. The prognosis was grim and negative. It was followed by a course of chemotherapy almost immediately and then further surgery. Within months the tumours were increasing and I began a course of radiotherapy. I was in a lot of pain, I had lost my appetite, I was having diarrhoea and I had very little stamina.

> *The doctors were amazed that my bone marrow and platelet counts and my immune system stayed so high.*

"Last September a friend suggested I take Essiac. After a few weeks, my appetite had returned and my weight increased. I sailed though a second course of chemotherapy despite warnings that some people couldn't tolerate that particular treatment and had to have transfusions. The doctors were amazed that my bone marrow and platelet counts and my immune system stayed so high. I have had no infections and feel quite energised. I am happy that I feel so well and I am very grateful for the tea."

Harlee Watson, UK, June 1998

"I was diagnosed with skin cancer in March 1997. I found a mole behind my left knee which was removed, together with some diseased blood tissue. The doctor wanted me to have some purely experimental tests which involved injecting some blue dye directly into the wound to see if the cancer had affected the lymph glands. I went home and thought about it and made a conscious decision there and then to stop all conventional treatment.

"I did not feel ill in the accepted sense but I realised that I had to do something for myself. At the time I was generally extremely run down. I had been neglecting myself and not caring about myself. To begin with I was in a blind panic about the cancer but to be honest the scare brought me to my senses.

I realised that I couldn't go on hating my physical body as much as I did and I can say now that I am glad that the cancer happened because it introduced me to Essiac, to something that 'walks its talk'.

"The information about the tea just fell into my lap as these things do. It was more the ideal behind what it was about that grabbed my interest at that time. For as long as I can remember I have had a problem with 'putting a price on healing'. To make money out of another's pain I find sickening but, when I say something about it, I am usually blasted with 'what about self worth?' So does self worth have to have a price?

"I have been taking Essiac for about seven months now, about four times a week. I feel better now than I have done for a very long time because now I am doing something useful. I'm telling people about the decoction and making it up for others. They are all coming back for more and they are all doing very well. One person is in remission, another is convinced the tumour is reduced and is fighting to have another scan to prove it."

Update (November 1998): "One man who started taking Essiac in April, having been pronounced inoperable, has been given the 'all clear'. The same is true of a woman who started with the tea in July. Yet another was given a month to live - three months ago"

D. O'Sullivan, UK, May 1998
"I was diagnosed with lung cancer in my left lung on 19th December 1997, undergoing surgery on 12th January 1998, which had to be abandoned due to the location of the carcinoma. Following this I had ten sessions of chemotherapy which left me weak and unable to swallow properly for quite a while. I heard about Essiac through friends and acquaintances and started taking the decoction on March 6th 1998.

"Within a period of six weeks my appetite had returned and my general health improved enormously. I weighed eight stones five pounds on February 12th and I weigh nine stones seven pounds today. Both the consultant at the hospital and my own doctor were amazed at the change in my appearance and at how well I looked. My doctor requested information about the tea for a retired doctor friend of his who is suffering from cancer of the colon.

> *Both the consultant at the hospital and my own doctor were amazed at the change in my appearance and at how well I looked.*

"August 1998:   It's six months since I had the operation and as of August 7th all my scans and tests are clear. The consultant told me that the tumour is fragmenting and he doesn't need to see me again. I have been taking Red Clover infusion during the day for the last three weeks as well as taking Essiac at night and I am feeling very well. I told the consultant that I walk three to four miles every day with my greyhound. He told me that I couldn't walk a quarter of a mile if that lung was packing up. He said I am looking extremely well and that I could come back and see him before Christmas if I wanted to but he was not going to scan me any more because he would just be filling me up with radium and I don't need that. He told me to go away for a holiday in Australia or New Zealand instead. The retired doctor told me he is doing very well on Essiac and is very pleased with the results."

David Vlastelica, UK, August 1998
Age 44
"I was diagnosed with metastasis in January 1998. The primary tumour on the kidney had produced a second tumour on my chest wall near the throat and a third in my right femur. The oncologist told me that there was nothing they could do for me because the cancer had already spread too far. They could only offer me palliative treatment when I would be needing it later. They put a nail down the centre of the femur to stabilise it and zapped it two months later with a single dose of radiotherapy. They offered me chemotherapy but I turned it down because they could only guarantee that it would make me feel awful.

"At the time of the visit to the oncologist, I was told that I had six months to live. I just would not accept this. I had done my research into the Essiac formula and decided to go with that. I have been taking it now for the past six months and I feel great. I'm working and that includes travelling between the UK and Central Europe and Canada and the United States.

"I had to make the first half-yearly appointment to see the oncologist again. He wouldn't do it because he was so convinced that I wouldn't be around to see him. He started laughing when I walked into his office three weeks ago.

"'You don't look ill,' he said. Then one of the other doctors came in.

"'Is this the guy who shouldn't be here?' he asked.

"Neither of them could explain why I was still around and looking very fit. I asked the oncologist how he would explain it if I was still around in another six months. He just shrugged and said, 'Then you didn't have cancer.'

"So if I die, I had cancer. If I live, despite the cancer-positive results of all the previous tests, I didn't have cancer. So who is in denial?"

L. Evans, UK, June 1998
"At Christmas last year I was thinking that I would lose my twelve-year-old Jack Russell terrier. She had had two heart attacks and was very poorly. I offered her Essiac and she licked up about a teaspoonful from my hand. I continued doing this for a week. As she wouldn't take a larger amount, I put 10ml in a measure and she did not object to me just putting it into her mouth.

"By March she was much more lively and eating well and now she does all the things she remembers doing when she was a puppy. For some years she had had a large lump on her rear end in an inoperable position. The veterinary surgeon says it's OK as long as it is not causing her any pain or becomes worse in any way. It has not improved since she has been taking the tea but it is not getting worse so we live in hope.

"For myself, having been a very fit seventy-eight-year-old, I was diagnosed as having high blood pressure and put on beta blockers etc. The tablets made me breathless and unable to do very much at all. Since taking Essiac I have regained a great deal of lost energy, I have cut down almost all of the tablets and my blood pressure averages 145/85. A friend of ours who takes Essiac as a tonic says it makes her sleep much better for the first time in years."

Since taking Essiac I have regained a great deal of lost energy.

D. Richmond, UK, July 1998 – *Age 53*
"I was diagnosed with multiple sclerosis (MS) in February 1991 after extensive tests, MRI scan, lumbar puncture, x-rays, etc. My neurologist said there was no treatment but if my symptoms {trembling limbs, body, head} worsened, I would have to have steroid treatment. I was not very happy.

"In August 1993 I was asked if I would like to try botulin injections into my neck every ten to twelve weeks – anything rather than steroids. Although this helped to stop my head shaking it didn't help the shaking limbs.

"In 1995, I started taking Essiac every night before retiring to bed and the tremors in all limbs ceased, with the exception of my left hand and arm. I continue to visit the neurologist but the amount of botulin he injects is half the original amount and he can't believe how well and calm I am. I have told him I take herbal tea. There isn't much of a comment but there again they don't scoff because they can see how well I am. I feel I am very lucky as I am able to work, I can drive and I can walk. I have a lovely, caring husband and family, and finally I can write because I am right-handed!"

Mali Klein, UK, June 1998
"My husband was supposed to be dead by Christmas 1993. Our diagnosis was brutally terminal after only eight months of marriage. A large and aggressive Glioblastoma Multiforme tumour growing on the site of my Vietnam veteran's old gun-

shot wound at the back of his head, seemed to be determined to give us a Christmas we didn't want. Greg started taking Essiac on December 7th 1993 and within a few days he was much steadier on his feet, his eyes came back into focus, he was out of bed and reading whole books again. I booked us a holiday in Iceland to see the New Year fireworks and then a place on the ferry to France.

"Greg's illness was directly related to the war wound he incurred in action in Vietnam in May 1967. The resulting hole in his skull relieved the pressure of the developing tumour on his brain to the point that it was already so large on diagnosis as to be completely inoperable and untreatable. Greg died May 11th 1994, with a sun tan and at home in the South of France, without 'tubes or morphine', pain-free and in awareness, exactly twenty-seven years to the day, all but fifteen hours, since he was so badly wounded in Vietnam. He was only fully comatose during the last four hours of his life and he died a wonderful death, absolutely on his own terms. He tolerated the high dose of steroid medication very well once he started taking Essiac. The continual discomfort when eating stopped almost immediately, he no longer needed a daily dose of laxatives and he maintained excellent energy and immune system levels, only becoming completely bedridden during the last twenty-four hours of life.

"The day before he died, his pulse and blood pressure readings were normal. The local doctor couldn't believe it when I called late the following evening, asking him to come and certify my husband's death. Unlike the majority of cancer patients, Greg did not die as a result of secondary infection caused by a weakening of the immune system. Death occurred when the pressure of the tumour on the brain stem caused sufficient deterioration in the vital functions governing breathing and the action of the heart. The bottles of morphine that he had been prescribed as a precaution were returned to the pharmacy with their seals unbroken.

"We know that the tea made a valuable contribution to both the quality of his life and to the nature of his death.

Apart from the inevitable facial swelling, he did not put on a lot of weight and we had fun until the day he died. He was cremated in the same clothes he had worn when we were married eighteen months before.

"I started drinking the tea in March 1994 as a tonic while I was nursing my husband and have taken it continually ever since as an experiment. I have to dilute the tea x 4 so as not to aggravate the scarring of a particularly nasty old duodenal ulcer that began life when I was sixteen, but my energy levels have remained high and I don't catch colds or 'flu. Most importantly for me, as someone who has been allergic to sucrose and fructose for many years, I am now able to eat most fruits and some dried fruit. Desserts are no longer 'just an apple' and candida is a thing of the past."

Rene Caisse at the Sub-Committee hearing in Bracebridge, February 1939:

"...*even the patients who died got relief from pain, and some of them had from eight months to two years comfortable life. I think I have letters from their families thanking me for the relief from pain, and the fact that these patients did not have to take narcotics before their death, and that they were conscious almost to the last, and seemed to be free from pain, and died in comfort.*"

L. Redford, ex-theatre nurse, UK, June 1998

"My cousin, aged thirty-four and with two small children, was diagnosed with malignant breast cancer in May 1997. The following month she underwent surgery involving a total mastectomy and lymphectomy. She was hoping to start chemotherapy and radiotherapy within a week but the wound would not heal. The nurses were changing the dressings every third day. They had tried everything, so after I had made up my cousin's next batch of Essiac, I wrapped the leftover herbs into a gauze wrap, like a poultice, and put it directly on to the wound. The effect was instantaneous. My cousin felt a sensation like having a tooth drawn and the pus began draining out of the wound. The district nurse brought some of the hospice nurses in to see it. They could hardly believe it but, within a couple of days, the wound was healed enough to consider chemotherapy.

"My cousin has taken Essiac continually for a year now and her health is steadily improving with each day. She holds great store by the tea and believes it has helped her immensely. She was the only one on her chemotherapy course who didn't need any changes in her cocktail of drugs, she had no nausea or vomiting and she did not lose her hair. A couple of weeks ago she did have a scare as she had begun to lose weight and discovered a swelling on her right side over her liver. After exhaustive tests she was given the all-clear with no signs of metastasis either in her liver, kidneys or gall bladder. Needless to say, she never misses her daily appointment with Nurse Caisse's wonderful legacy."

She was the only one on her chemotherapy course who didn't need any changes in her cocktail of drugs, she had no nausea or vomiting and she did not lose her hair.

Sheep sorrel Planting Trials

Trial One

Site: an established, organically controlled vegetable garden in Southern England, semi-shaded early morning, late afternoon.

Plot size: 1 metre/39ins square

Soil type: good loam

Ph: neutral to acidic

Situation: Sheep sorrel plants in second year of active growth, having been raised from seed the previous year. Young plants thinned when dormant the previous winter, roots dried, powdered and stored.

Objective: To harvest leaves and stems just prior to full flowering.

First cut: May 9th 1998

Yield:

Wet weight: 1lb 13 ozs/822g

Dry weight: 3.24ozs/92g

Second cut: June 10th 1998

Yield

Wet weight: 5lbs/2.268g

Dry weight: 8.5ozs/240g

Third cut: July 30th 1998

Yield

Wet weight: 1lb 14ozs/850g

Dry weight: 3.35ozs/95g

Plants rested and allowed to seed.

Summary

Total annual yield:

Wet weight: 8lbs 11ozs/3940g

Dry weight: 15ozs/427g

Conclusion: A minimum of 5 people taking 30ml daily of the decoction can be supplied with Sheep sorrel for a period of up to fifteen months from a plot 1 metre square.

Trial Two

Site: Adjacent to Trial One.

Plot size: 1 metre/39ins square

Soil type + ph value, light availability identical to Trial One

Objective: To grow Sheep sorrel from seed and to test availability and yield during the same season.

Seed sown: March 20th 1998.

Germination time: Four weeks

First cut: August 1st 1998

Yield:

Wet weight: 2lb 14 ozs/1304g

Dry weight: 4.23ozs/120g

Plants rested and allowed to seed.

Summary

Total annual yield:

Wet weight: 2lbs 14ozs/1304g

Dry weight: 4.23ozs/120g

Conclusion: Within 4 months after germination from seed, the plants from a plot 1 metre square will supply 1 person taking 30ml daily + 1 person taking 15 ml daily of the decoction with Sheep sorrel sufficient for a period of up to fifteen months.

Glossary of Terms

alterative Tending to alter or produce alteration, as in tending to restore normal health.

antioxidant Compound or substance that inhibits oxidation.

antispasmodic Compound or substance that eases or prevents spasms.

astringent A term describing the binding action of many herbal remedies on mucous membranes and exposed tissues, providing an impenetrable barrier to most infective organisms and many toxins.

beta blockers Any of a group of drugs used to treat abnormal heart conditions and high blood pressure. They slow down the action of the heart by blocking the action of nerve endings known as beta receptors.

botulin Any of several nerve toxins produced by the bacterium, *Clostridium botulinum*, found in improperly smoked or canned foods.

carcinoma Any of a large variety of malignant tumours derived from epithelial cells covering the surface of a tissue.

cell proliferant A substance that acts to reproduce or produce new cells rapidly and repeatedly.

decoction A preparation made by boiling remedies in water.

demulcents Remedies that are primarily soothing in effect, characteristically serving to enhance associated healing or astringent properties.

diaphoretic Inducing perspiration.

diuretic A substance that causes an increased output of urine.

douche Washing out a body cavity or opening by a stream of water or other fluid

enema The introduction of liquid into the rectum for therapeutic purposes

expectorant A substance that assists in the removal of sticky mucoid sputum from the bronchial tubes.

glioblastoma multiforme Astrocytoma grade IV. Diffusely invasive of normal brain cells, so tumour cells are usually left behind during surgery.

glucoside A specific sugar related to a product of glucose.

glycoside A term generally applied to compounds of all sugars.

husbandry (good) The careful management of resources relating to the cultivation of plants or the raising of livestock.

infusion A preparation made by steeping remedies in hot water.

metastasis The migration of tumour cells away from a primary tumour, usually by way of the bloodstream or lymph fluid, to another site in the body to initiate a secondary tumour or tumours.

mucilage Slimy fluids containing the complex carbohydrate constituents of many plants, acting as demulcent and soothing agents with associated healing effects.

oxalate Any salt or ester of oxalic acid.

refrigerant As having cooling or fever-reducing properties.

relaxant As inducing muscle relaxation or relieving tension.

steroid drugs A large group of synthetic drugs; those specific to cancer palliative care are generally prescribed to relieve inflammation and oedema.

synergy The action of two or more substances, organs or organisms to achieve an effect greater than the sum of their individual effects.

Resources and Suppliers

UK

For up-to-date information on herbal suppliers:

The Herb Society,
(Registered Charity No 265511)
Deddington Hill Farm,
Warmington,
Banbury, OX17 1XB
Tel: 01295 692000

The Nat Inst of Medical Herbalists
56 Longbrook Street
Exeter, EX4 6AH
Tel: 01392 426022

The British Herbal Medicine Association
Sun House, Church Street,
Stroud, Glos. GL5 1JL
Tel: 01453 751389

SEEDS:

John Chambers' Wild Flower Seeds
15 Westleigh Rd, Barton Seagrave,
Kettering, Northants. NN15 5AJ
Tel: 01933 652562
(for supplies of Sheep sorrel and Burdock seed)

ORGANIC HERBS:

Hambledon Herbs
Court Farm, Milverton,
Som. TA4 1NF
Tel: 01823 401 205
(for buying herbs <u>individually</u>)

KOMBUCHA:

Kombucha Supplies UK
The Hollies, Mill Hill,
Wellow, Bath, BA2 8QJ
Tel: 01225 833150;
Fax: 01225 840012
(and for all Kombucha brewing needs)

SPIRULINA:

Xynergy Health Products
Unit 6b, Old Station Yard,
Elsted, Midhurst,
W. Sussex GU29 0JT
Tel: 01730-813642
in powder and tablet form

ESSIAC INFORMATION:

The Clouds Trust
(Registered Charity No 1064289),
P.O.Box 30, Liss, Hants., GU33 7XF
e-mail: cloudsadmin@onet.co.uk
web:http://home.onet.co.uk/~cloudstrust
For copies of all Clouds Trust leaflets and
A Future Beyond the Sun by Mali Klein

Canada

New Action Products,
P.O.Box 141, Grimsby, Ont. L3M 4G5
Tel: 716 662 8000

"THE RENE CAISSE STORY" (Video)

For a copy of the only film record of
Rene Caisse in existence:
Call Toll Free 1 888 773 7973
or visit the website:
http://www.muskoka.com/caisse

USA

HERBS:

Blessed Herbs,
109 Barre Plains Road,
Oakham, MA 01068
Tel: 508 882 3839

Herb Research Foundation
Box 2602, Longmont, CO 80501, USA
Tel: 303 449 2265

New Action Products,
Box 540, Orchard Park, NY 14127
Tel: 1 800 541 3799

Australia

For all enquiries re: herbal suppliers:
National Herbalists Association of Australia
49 Oakwood Street, Sutherland, NSW 2232, Australia
Tel: 02 92 116 437

An SAE with all enquiries would be appreciated

Bibliography

Bartholomew, A. & M., *Kombucha Tea for Your Health and Healing*, Gateway, 1998
Belkin, M & Fitzgerald, D, *Tumour Damaging Capacity of Plant Materials*, National Cancer Institute Journal, 1952
Cadenas, Enrique & Lester Packer, *Handbook of Antioxidants*, Dekker, 1996
Caisse, Rene M., RN, *"I was Canada's Cancer Nurse"*, The Story of Essiac, 1963
The Canadian Journal of Herbalism, Vol.12, No.3, July 1991
Castleman, Michael, *The Healing Herbs*, Rodale Press, PA, 1991
Christopher, Dr. John R., *The School of Natural Healing*, 1976
Clapham, Tutin & Moore, *Flora of the British Isles*, 3rd ed., 1987
Debo, Angie, *A History of the Indians of the United States*, Pimlico ed., Random, 1995
Department of Resources and Development, *Native Trees of Canada*, 4th ed., 1950
Ericsen-Brown, Charlotte, *Use of Plants for the Past Five Hundred Years*, 1979
Fisher, John, *The Origins of Garden Plants*, Constable, London
Grimm, W.C., *The Book of Trees*, 1957
Grieve, Maude, *A Modern Herbal*, Vols. 1&2, 1982
Herbal Research Publications Inc., *Naturopathic Handbook of Herbal Formulas*, 1995
Hutchens, Alma R., *Indian Herbology of North America*, Shambhala Publications, 1973
Henrikson, Robert, *Earth Food Spirulina*, 1997
Hodgkinson, A. *Oxalic Acid in Biology and Medicine*, Academic Press, 1977
Hoffmann, David, *The Herbal Handbook*, 1987
Jackson & Teague, *Handbook of Alternatives to Chemical Medicine*, 1975
Klein, Mali, *A Future Beyond the Sun*, Fisher Miller, 1997
Kloss, Jethro, *Back to Eden*, Woodbridge Press, 1972
Kramer & Koslowski, *Physiology of Woody Plants*, Academic Press, 1979
Kretovich, V.L., *Principles of Plant Biochemistry*, Pergamon Press, 1966
Kruger, Anna, *Herbs*, American Nature Guides, 1992
Launett, Edwin, *Hamlyn Guide to Edible & Medicinal Plants Britain & N. Europe*
Lust, John, *The Herb Book*, Bantam Books, 1974.
Meyer, J.E., *The Herbalist*, 1976.
Mills, *Out of the Earth: The Essential Book of Herbal Medicine*, Viking, 1991
Mills, Simon, *The Dictionary of Modern Herbalism*, Thorsons, 1985
Mills, Simon, *The Complete Guide to Modern Herbalism*, Thorsons, 1994
Moss, Ralph, *Cancer Therapy*, 1992
Mowrey, Daniel B., *The Scientific Validation of Herbal Medicine*, 1986
Ministry of Natural Resources, Canada, *The Forest Trees of Ontario*, 1986
Nature Trek Guide, *Wild Herbs of Britain and Europe*
Raven, Evert & Eichhorn, *Biology of Plants*, 5th ed., 1992
Readers Digest, The Beauty and Splendour of North America
Readers Digest, North American Folk Healing, 1998
Shook, Dr Edward E., *Advanced Treatise on Herbology*, 1934
Snow, Sheila, *The Essence of Essiac*, 1993
Snow, Sheila, *Old Ontario Remedies*, *"Rene Caisse, Essiac"*
Snow & Allen, *"Could Essiac Halt Cancer?"*, Homemakers, July 1977
Snow, Sheila & Klein, Mali, *The Rene Caisse Formula Interview*, 1996
Steen, Dr R. Grant, *A Conspiracy of Cells, The Basic Science of Cancer*, Plenum, 1993
Stuart, Malcolm, *The Encyclopaedia of Herbs and Herbalism*, 1987
Tierra, Michael, *Planetary Herbology*, Lotus Press, 1988
Tierra, Michael, *The Way of Herbs*, Pocket Books, 1983.
Thain, M, & M. Hickman, *Penguin Book of Biology*, 1996
US Congress, Office of Technology Assessment, *Unconventional Cancer Treatment*, Washington DC, 1990
USA Today, *"The Great Elm Returns"*, November 6th 1997
Watt & Brandwijk, *Medicinal & Poisonous Plants of S & E Africa*, Livingston, 1962
Weiner, Michael A. & Janet, *Herbs that Heal*, 1994
Williams, Penny, *"New Frontiers"*, Homemakers Magazine, October 1995
Youngson, Robert M., Collins Dictionary of Medicine, 1992

Index